T0195361

NAVIGATING HEALTHCARE REFORM

AN INSIDER'S GUIDE FOR NURSES AND ALLIED HEALTH PROFESSIONALS

NAVIGATING HEALTHCARE REFORM

AN INSIDER'S GUIDE FOR NURSES AND ALLIED HEALTH PROFESSIONALS

Peter Edelstein, MD
Chief Medical Officer
Elsevier Clinical Solutions

ELSEVIER

ELSEVIER

3251 Riverport Lane
St. Louis, Missouri 63043

NAVIGATING HEALTHCARE REFORM: AN INSIDER'S GUIDE FOR
NURSES AND OTHER HEALTH PROFESSIONALS   ISBN: 978-0-323-52977-8

International Standard Book Number: 978-0-323-52977-8

Executive Content Strategist: Lee Henderson
Senior Content Development Manager: Laurie Gower
Senior Content Development Specialist: Laura Goodrich
Publishing Services Manager: Julie Eddy
Senior Project Manager: Mary G. Stueck
Design Direction: Ryan Cook

Printed in the United States of America

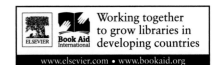

Working together
to grow libraries in
developing countries

www.elsevier.com • www.bookaid.org

Last digit is the print number: 9 8 7 6 5 4 3 2 1

*This work is dedicated with the deepest appreciation
to all of the nurses and health professionals who,
over the years, stayed up into the wee hours
to teach me how to care for our patients…*

Acknowledgments

With special thanks to my dear friend, *Michelle R. Troseth, MSN, RN, DPNAP, FAAN*, a true pioneer in translating strategic visions of Interprofessional Healthcare into meaningful patient care at the bedside. Michelle honors me (and greatly benefits you) by having co-authored the superb chapter on *Interprofessional Education and Collaborative Care* found within this book.

Peter Edelstein, MD

Contributors

Tracy Christopherson, PhD(c), MS, BAS, RRT
Boyne City, Michigan

Michelle R. Troseth, MSN, RN, DPNAP, FAAN
Chief Professional Practice Officer
Elsevier Clinical Solutions

Reviewers

Michelle Acorn, DNP, NP, PHC/Adult, BA, BScN/PHCNP, MN/ACNP, ENC(C), GNC(C), CGP, CAP
Doctor of Nurse Practitioner, Primary Health Care
Global Health Nurse Practitioner Coordinator
Nursing Department
University of Toronto
Toronto, Ontario
Canada

Abimbola Farinde, PhD, PharmD
Professor
School of Nursing and Health Sciences
Columbia Southern University
Orange Beach, Alabama

Penny Fauber, RN, BSN, MS, PhD
Director Practical Nursing Department

Natalie Fischetti, RN, PhD
Associate Professor
Nursing Department
College of Staten Island
City University of New York
New York, New York

Jane Clifford O'Brien, PhD, OTR/L, FAOTA
Professor
Occupational Therapy
University of New England
Portland, Maine

Sherry Lynn Hobgood Pomeroy, RN, PhD
Professor Emerita, School of Nursing,
University at Buffalo, The State University of New York
New York, New York;
Senior Lecturer, Niagara University, School of Nursing
Niagara County, New York;
Faith Community Nurse
Orchard Park Presbyterian Church
Orchard Park, New York

Elizabeth A. Summers, MSN, RN, CNE
Coordinator of Practical Nurse Program
Cass Career Center
Harrisonville, Missouri

Stephen F. Wehrman, RRT, RPFT
Professor Emeritus
Department of Health Sciences
Kapi'olani Community College
Honolulu, Hawaii

Suzanne White, MSN, RN, PHCNS-BC
Associate Professor
Nursing Department
Morehead State University
Morehead, Kentucky

Foreword

I will never forget the first time that I watched Peter give a presentation. I was amazed, hooked, and totally focused. Everyone in the audience of the Elsevier Leadership Forum in 2014 was equally as rapt. It was an intimate setting with many health professions, but primarily nurses. He walked on stage in his business suit and immediately began undressing; fortunately, he stopped when he reached his second-layer of clothing, his surgical attire. The audience was both shocked and relieved at the same time, laughing in response. He had transformed from the businessman to the surgeon, the great Dr. Edelstein. When he finished speaking, I immediately wanted him to share with the members of my team the evolution that he presented. I enjoyed the presentation again and, to tell you the truth, I would enjoy seeing it again today. I know that he would provide us with new discoveries.

In Peter's terms, I am a lay person, although I have experience with health accreditation as it is the primary focus of the Accrediting Bureau of Health Education Schools. Our staff works with many subject matter experts in healthcare as we have evaluated every type of program that one might imagine. We have about 1,500 programs that are reviewed annually.

So, I believe that Peter floated his idea by me for no other reason than the evolution of the health world we are seeing as we work with health professions as well as credentialing bodies. Or maybe it was because something presented a beautiful image in his mind of health tumbling in an out of what he knew as medicine . . . way back when.

As we navigate the many models of today's platform, collaboration is a requirement with the ever-changing dynamics of health care. Peter—then and now—continues to discuss industry-validated learning experiences and how they apply to both nurses and allied health professionals in practice.

Florence Tate
Executive Director
Accrediting Bureau of Health Education Schools

Contents

CHAPTER 1

Welcome Aboard

Why Would a Physician Author a Book for Nurses and Allied Health Professionals?

Many people will naturally—perhaps cynically—ask why a *physician* (and a *surgeon,* of all things) authored a practical guide on navigating healthcare reform for *nurses and allied health professionals.* Perhaps a (true) anecdote from early in my own surgical training will best explain my perspective that the optimal approach to caring for patients should be highly collaborative and broadly interprofessional.

It was my first night on call as a surgical intern. Only 5 days earlier, I had proudly received my medical degree. *I was a doctor. A physician.* And *I knew absolutely nothing of real value or practicality about patient care.* Thus it was with overwhelming trepidation that I answered my first page (we had "beepers" back then) on my first night of call as a physician. I had been assigned as the intern "slave" to the cardiac surgery service, knowing little more than that the heart was not heart shaped and that it pumped blood from somewhere within the chest. The phone call was from my frantic Surgical Fellow (whom I had yet to meet), now in his ninth year of training and the last of 3 years focused exclusively on cardiac surgery.

"Are you my new idiot intern?" he demanded. (Clearly, surgical training was to be warm and nurturing.)

Trying not to darken the crotch of my greens, I stammered, "Ye–yes."

He explained at warp speed that a patient who had undergone open heart surgery earlier in the day was bleeding into his chest, likely the result of a ruptured suture line. (Upon hearing this, I think I might have temporarily passed out. . . .) The Surgical Fellow went on to frantically explain that if I "didn't get my intern ass to the cardiac ICU and open the man's chest pronto, *the patient will die!*"

In a daze, I ran the unfamiliar hallways until I stumbled into the cardiac intensive care unit (ICU). As the doors automatically swooshed open, I hesitantly shuffled in.

This was an old Veterans Administration (VA) hospital, and the nurse who immediately deconstructed me with an experienced, critical eye appeared to have begun her healthcare career during the Civil War. She knew everything about ICU cardiac care, and I knew nothing. And she knew it, and I knew it.

In retrospect, this was a pivotal moment that engendered within me the complete belief in a collaborative, interprofessional team approach to patient care (a foundational professional philosophy that remains deeply embedded within me to this day).

"You must be Dr. Edelstein," she stated in a voice that was quiet, stern, and steady but absent of all criticism or judgment.

"Must I be?" I asked, only half joking.

"I understand that you're here to open this patient's chest to prevent him from imminent death as a result of cardiac tamponade." (In cardiac tamponade, blood fills the sac surrounding the heart, rapidly restricting the heart's ability to pump blood.)

"Yes, ma'am," I said in a trembling voice.

She led a reluctant me to the man's bedside as she spoke.

"I've taken the opportunity to prep the patient's chest and lay out all of the instruments that you might need, Doctor." Again, she spoke without a touch of sarcasm or superiority as she pointed to a table with an array of sterile surgical instruments at the ready.

"Yes, ma'am," I repeated as I reached for one which, like all of the shiny tools laid out before me, appeared entirely alien.

"I'm certain, Dr. Edelstein, that you wish to begin this emergency procedure with the *sternal wire cutters,*" she said calmly, pointing to an instrument far from the one for which I was reaching.

"Yes, ma'am," I said, now shakily picking up the instrument to which she had directed my hand.

"And I am sure, Doctor, that you'll wish to *immediately begin by cutting all of the sternal wires,* starting from the superior aspect of the surgical incision, to release the pressure from the blood building up around the patient's heart."

"Yes, ma'am," I whispered as I cut the wires, and blood gushed onto the patient's chest, bed sheets, and me.

"Well done, Doctor," she said with sincere praise, as we both looked up at the monitor to witness the sudden rise in the man's blood pressure to viable levels.

Just then, the Surgery Fellow rushed into the ICU, yelling for the nurse.

"Everything's fine, Doctor," the nurse said in a authoritative tone as the panicked Fellow raced to the bedside. "Dr. Edelstein has done an excellent job of saving your patient."

The Fellow may have nodded to me (doubtful), and, along with the nurse, he rapidly pushed the patient's bed out of the ICU toward the operating room. I collapsed in a chair, my limbs rubber. My gloves and greens were covered in blood (the patient's) and sweat (mine). After about 10 minutes, the nurse returned and began stoically gathering the instruments I had used.

"You . . ." I stammered. *"You saved him."*

"No, Doctor," she replied. *"You saved him. By allowing me to show you how."*

She looked me up and down. "If you want to be a truly good doctor, allow me to give you some advice."

I waited in silence, anxious for any pearls of wisdom that would help me to survive the remainder of this call night, let alone my career.

"Over the next couple of years, as you care for patients on the wards and here in the ICU, there will be few if any situations or procedures that you'll understand better than I do. I am an expert in critical care medicine. So if you do as well as you did tonight, if you listen respectfully and graciously, the good nurses and pharmacists and therapists and technicians *will teach you*. . . even befriend you."

I nodded solemnly.

"And if you let us teach you, not only will you get more sleep," (and here she smiled for the first time, a small, mischievous smile), "your patients will do better. *Much better.*"

"But," I asked, "how will I repay you?"

"You're here for what, 7 years?"

I nodded. After this first call night's initial adventure, 7 years stretched out ahead of me like 7 decades.

"A couple of years from now, you'll leave us and begin your life in the operating room. You'll see and do things that we never get to see or understand. We'll only see your patients after you've rebuilt their insides. So here's the deal: *we'll teach you now, you teach us then*. Explain the diseases. Draw me pictures of what you did in the OR and why. Help me be better at my job like I helped you be better at your job tonight."

Then she smiled again, this time warmly. "Deal?"

"Deal," I replied with a grin.

Throughout my career as a surgeon and educator, the lesson I first learned that night at the hands of a wise, old VA nurse, the power of *collaborative, interprofessional patient care*, has proven its worth to me time and time again, both subtly and overtly. I am a passionate believer in *placing the patient at the center of all care* (with the patient and his or her loved ones serving as major participants in care decisions). Joining me and surrounding that patient are scores of clinical care providers. And now it seems that the focus on patient-centered and interprofessional care have at last begun moving slowly toward center stage as the philosophical stars of the US healthcare system.

> The focus on patient-centered and interprofessional care have at last begun moving slowly toward center stage as the philosophical stars of the US healthcare system.

And finally, I wrote this book because, simply said, I like the kind of people who devote themselves to serving patients. I have always enjoyed both professionally and personally working alongside dedicated nurses, therapists, technicians, dieticians, and other healthcare providers because we are all committed to caring for those in need, each of us helping via different but partially overlapping skills, experiences, and perspectives.

These are the reasons why a physician wrote a guide for nurses and allied health professionals. And before we continue, a bit of housekeeping: terminology in healthcare is constantly evolving. Thus some use the term "allied health professionals," whereas others prefer "health professionals." In this guide, we will use the latter. Along with allied health professionals, this book is written for nurses, pharmacists, and other healthcare providers, both students and practitioners, in the sincere hope that you benefit from my musings.

I thank you for picking up my work. And now I encourage you to read and reread the practical information offered in the following chapters as you navigate the ever-changing waters of healthcare reform and, in doing so, you attempt to best serve your patients and yourself.

In the Eye of the Storm

Monster waves. Fierce winds. Crashing lightning. Roaring thunder

We are sailing through the eye of a violent storm. A storm the likes of which our US healthcare system has never before experienced, let alone successfully navigated. Until literally just a few years ago, the practice of healthcare in the United States had basically flowed gently along for decades. For centuries, really. Ours was an extremely simple care delivery model, easy for all to understand and participate in. Doctors were doctors. Nurses were nurses. Patients were patients. Those providing care did their best, their expertise and outcomes rarely challenged. And those receiving care demonstrating unreserved appreciation, paying what they could in precious metals, goods, or services.

Of course, there were some small waves and brief gusts over the decades, as some mild, rolling changes worked their way through healthcare. Insurance companies, both private and government (**Medicare, Medicaid,** and similar state programs), replaced the patient and family as the source of direct reimbursement to care providers (and insurers tended to pay in cash rather than in gold dust or chickens). And there was consistent expansion in the number and variety of care specialists (physician, nurse, and health professional), so that today, we have physical and occupational and respiratory and speech therapists, numerous levels of nurses, a variety of assistants, and technicians of all kinds. And over time, the independent doctor and nurse frequently joined the growing population of allied health professionals who had economically aligned themselves with (or were even employed by) specific hospitals, clinics, or healthcare networks. And of course, just as darkness follows light, medical malpractice attorneys began to creep out of the legal shadows (just kidding … sort of), and malpractice litigation began to influence healthcare, driving providers and hospitals to practice financially costly "defensive medicine" (a predictable response to an overly litigious society). Still, even with these significant waves and gusts rocking and rolling the healthcare ship, the basic practice and model of healthcare delivery in the United States remained as it had always been: doctors were the captains of the ship, continuing to serve as the dominant decision makers and focus of healthcare; nurses, therapists, pharmacists, technicians, and other allied health professionals were members of the crew, serving the captains as "physician extenders"; patients were largely viewed as cargo, on the periphery of their own care decisions; the captains' care plans and treatment outcomes remained both unquestioned and unrelated to reimbursement; and healthcare costs were rarely if ever openly discussed.

Then, seemingly overnight (to those of us with gray hair or, in my case, little hair), we sailed directly into the heart of the healthcare reform storm. But in truth, dark, threatening clouds had been visible on the horizon for years. We had just refused to see them until we could no longer avoid slamming into the maelstrom. Suddenly, US healthcare began rapidly transforming into something virtually unrecognizable. And *irreversible* (although multiple iterations of the current form are likely over the upcoming years). Now we are faced with new, gale force winds in the form of *quality requirements, regulations, improvement processes, cost-efficiency goals,* and *buzzwords*. ***Value-based Reimbursement. Population***

Health Management. Accountable Care Organizations and *Patient-Centered Medical Homes. Meaningful Use. Patient Engagement. The Triple Aim. CPOE* and *EHRs* and *PQRS* and the *ACA* and a whole litany of other alphabetical acronyms threatening to sink our ship.

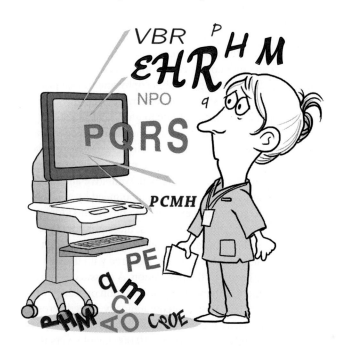

OK, enough of the nautical analogies. I don't want to go *overboard*.

Today's US healthcare reform does not represent an *evolution* in healthcare delivery. It is a *revolution*. Not only in how we view healthcare but in *how we view health*. In how we both as an industry and a society understand the roles and responsibilities not only of physicians but also of nurses and nurse practitioners, physical therapists, dieticians, medical assistants, pharmacy technicians, social workers, administrators. And *patients*.

Today's US healthcare reform does not represent an *evolution* in healthcare delivery. It is a *revolution*. Not only in how we view healthcare, but in *how we view health*.

Truly our entire traditional healthcare philosophy and model are being turned on their heads. Although the US healthcare system is leading the way, we are far from alone. Dynamic changes in healthcare are slowly (and not so slowly) spreading across the rest of the world, driven by spiraling healthcare costs, epidemics of conditions and diseases, shortages of care providers, and aging and growing populations. Some countries' healthcare philosophies and models are similar enough to ours that they are aiming to learn from "what the United States is doing right" and "what the United States is doing wrong" in hopes of saving their nations time and money (and political angst); examples include Australia, the United Kingdom, and the United Arab Emirates. But to those in other countries, the traditional US healthcare system was already foreign in philosophy and design prior to recent reform. Still struggling to provide basic needs to massive populations that continue to grow, and limited by few physicians and a paucity of advanced care centers, many developing countries (especially in Africa and Asia) are faced with seemingly unassailable healthcare obstacles. In some, care delivery challenges (especially preventative and out-of-hospital maintenance care) are compounded by a general lack of respect (sometimes even among physicians) for nurses and allied health professionals; these providers are not viewed as true clinicians and, therefore, are not appreciated as a significant, available provider resource with the power to improve the health of the population. A classic example is Indonesia, the fourth most populous nation on Earth, with over 260,000,000 inhabitants geographically spread across 17,000 islands. There are far too many people for far too few physicians (roughly one doctor per 10,000 people, versus 23 per 10,000 in the United States and 22 per 10,000 in the United Kingdom)[1] spread out far too widely. But there is little respect for and belief in care providers other than physicians; thus, the nation has yet to tap into the reserve of nurses and allied health professionals who could be further trained to provide impactful care to the massive population. For Indonesia and many other poor, heavily populated nations with such different philosophies and models, closely following the successes and failures of the current US approach to healthcare reform offers only limited potential benefit.

But although healthcare reform is truly a global issue, in this guidebook we will be focusing on healthcare reform in the United States. We will review the critical factors that are driving reform, including:

- *Financial,* as the healthcare spend (both direct and indirect) already represents a massive portion of the US economy and is continuing to outpace inflation[2]
- *Operational,* in which the demand for integrated inpatient and outpatient acute care, long-term care, home care,

physical therapy, occupational therapy, pharmaceutical consultation, and medication compliance is creating ever more complex challenges

- *Personal,* because in no other industry is every living human being either currently or guaranteed-to-someday-be a consumer (i.e., a patient).

However, the goal of this work is not simply *to understand* the basic drivers of today's US healthcare reform. We will build such a foundational understanding because it is necessary to achieve the true purpose of this book: *to help guide you as you navigate your professional career through this actively changing healthcare delivery environment.* And we need you to do more than simply successfully navigate healthcare reform. *We need you to lead healthcare reform* as we strive for consistent, sustainable, high-quality, cost-efficient, preventative, and out-of-hospital maintenance care (that's a mouthful!). Because the math alone tells us that without nurses and allied health professionals leading the charge, we will fall far short before realizing meaningful reform:

- There are more than 325,000,000 patients and future patients spread across this great nation.
- There are only 442,000 primary care physicians and 484,000 specialist physicians (that is one primary care physician for every 735 Americans)[3].
- Unlike the general population, physicians still overwhelmingly cluster around urban centers (geographic asymmetry, meaning that many current and future patients live in rural regions where the ratio of patients to physician is far greater, especially to specialty and subspecialty physicians)[4].
- There are almost 3,200,000 registered nurses in the United States and 827,000 licensed practical nurses[5].
- Allied health professionals? Unbelievable! By 2020 there will be an estimated *19.8 million* working in our country![6]

Here are some more numbers to support my conclusion. These statistics are from the US Department of Labor (DOL). The DOL publishes a list of projected rankings for "The Fastest Growing Occupations" from 2014 through 2024.[7] Here are some notable rankings:

- #2 is occupational therapy assistants
- #3? physical therapist assistants
- #4? physical therapist aides
- Home health aides? #5

- Nurse practitioners are #7 (you guessed it…right after commercial divers)
- Next are physical therapists
- At #10, after statisticians, are ambulance drivers and attendants.

So 7 of the top 10 fastest growing occupations in the United States are nurses and allied health professionals or healthcare related. In fact, *over the next decade, 20 of the 30 occupations projected to grow most rapidly are nurses and allied health professionals or healthcare related,* including:

- Physician assistants
- Genetic counselors
- Audiologists
- Diagnostic medical sonographers
- Phlebotomists
- Nursing midwives
- Emergency medical technicians
- Paramedics
- Optometrists

This massive wake of nursing and health professional career opportunities represents the huge wake trailing the US healthcare ship as it sails headlong into reform (sorry… couldn't keep away from the nautical analogies). The DOL data support the conclusion that without the addition to our workforce of tens of thousands of new nurses, pharmacy technicians, physician assistants, respiratory therapists, and dozens and dozens of other healthcare professionals (not to mention social workers, case workers, translators, shuttle drivers, administrators, etc.), we will fall far short of our reform goals. And note this: many reform "goals" are more than goals, they are *economic necessities* and, in a final nod to sailors, failure to achieve significant healthcare reform will sink the US economy.

So, there you have it. The math doesn't lie. Even if they had the time and temperament, the limited number of US physicians would never be able to serve as the sole leaders for today and tomorrow's massive and complex healthcare reform activities while still providing medical and surgical care to their patients.

In the end, we're left with this: Today's healthcare reform represents *The Age of Nursing and Allied Health Professionals.*

What do I mean? That for the nation to (1) truly achieve consistent, sustainable, high-quality, cost-efficient healthcare and (2) for our population to move from reactive, acute, inpatient care to proactive, out-of-hospital, preventative, and maintenance care, *healthcare reform must be led* by the ranks of registered nurses, respiratory therapists, diagnostic medical sonographers, licensed practical nurses, dieticians, and dozens and dozens of additional care specialists spanning the healthcare delivery continuum.

Today's healthcare reform represents The Age of Nursing and Allied Health Professionals.

And embracing this powerful potential army of care providers demands that *we further invest in you*: in your additional training aimed at *expanding your clinical knowledge and activities and patient care responsibilities.*

About This Book

This book is not meant to be a tome, an exhaustive review, or an introspective study of today's healthcare reform. In fact, quite the opposite. It is meant to be a *practical guide for nurses, therapists, technicians, assistants, and other allied health professionals, providing a clear, rapid, and succinct understanding of the critical themes that underlie today's shifting healthcare environment.* As such, this work is created for both student and practitioner alike because these are key concepts and critical issues you will repeatedly encounter at many points along your healthcare career path.

Throughout the chapters, you'll find words in **bold print.** These selected words will join other commonly used terms in the Glossary at the end of the text. Refer to the Glossary to refresh your memory whenever you run into a vaguely recalled multiletter acronym or healthcare reform buzzword (which will happen all the time, believe me).

Throughout each chapter, you'll find an image of a pearl ⬤ and the word "**Pearl,**" short for *"Clinical Pearls."* Well known among medical students and physicians, *Pearls* are critical summary points, synoptic knowledge to be remembered and referred to in your daily activities and throughout your career.

This book is designed to be used however you wish; that is, you can read it from cover to cover, or you can selectively target chapters or sections for reading and repeated reference. Finally, if you find the book of no practical value, I've been told that it works fairly well to start a campfire.

● **PEARL**

- After decades of traditional healthcare, we are in the midst of truly disruptive reform aimed at achieving *consistent, sustainable, high-quality, cost-efficient care.*
- Today's reform revolution is not just about healthcare, it is also about *health.*
- Healthcare reform aims to move us from the reactive, acute, inpatient care model to *proactive, out-of-hospital, preventative, and maintenance care.*
- Although the current healthcare reform will likely be repeatedly modified over time, *the foundational concepts and drivers of the reform revolution are here to stay.*
- *Unless nurses and allied health professionals not only participate in, but lead, reform activities,* consistent, sustainable, high-value healthcare will never be fully realized.

In each chapter, you'll find *"Pearls"*: critical summary points and synoptic knowledge to be remembered and referred to in your daily activities and throughout your career.

Last but not least, this book is not meant to be a referendum on today's healthcare reform legislation or on the political motives or specific individuals involved in this hotly debated issue. The likely reality is that healthcare reform, albeit likely modified in form in the future, is here to stay. Regardless of Supreme Court challenges and changing administrations, the foundational issues that have brought us to this point are not going to simply correct themselves or fade away. And the founding principles that have led us to today's reform, as we will discuss, offer us the opportunity to drive cost reduction (i.e., cost-of-care efficiencies) by consistently and sustainably providing high-quality healthcare.

So There You Have It...

Now you have some insight into my motives in authoring a healthcare reform guide specifically for nurses and allied health professionals.

As for goals, I have two. First, I hope that this book will be of benefit as you search for professional satisfaction. *Seek out opportunities* to learn more, to advance your clinical knowledge and skills. Don't shy away, but *seize new responsibilities*. Rather than wait for it to be offered, *ask to lead*. And remember, none of this has to be on a grand scale. I don't expect (or encourage) a recent graduate in physical therapy to demand the position of hospital Chief Executive Officer. But any care provider can have a good idea; offer a better approach; model high-quality, compassionate care. Leading in activities and improvement processes for your patients, on your ward, across your service line, and in your care setting can dramatically and favorably impact patients and their families, as well as other providers with whom you work. So *do it*.

But professional satisfaction alone is not what primarily led many of us (perhaps most of us) to seek a healthcare career. (And it certainly wasn't the money—internet celebrities have demonstrated that there are far faster ways that require much less—if any—effort or talent to reap in piles of cash.) Training and practicing as a nurse, physical therapist, speech therapist, physician assistant, pharmacy tech, or for any one of the many other care provider roles is both demanding and exhausting (emotionally and physically). For us, healthcare is not a job, it's a *calling*. Because, as corny as it sounds, we chose a patient care career because *we like to help people*. So the second goal of this guide is to help you find roles and responsibilities that allow you to experience *personal fulfillment* as a patient care provider.

Thus I challenge you to view today's healthcare reform revolution, as unstable and unpredictable as it is, as *an opportunity to elevate and achieve your professional and personal goals, dreams, and successes.*

References

1. *NationMaster.* 2002–2003 data. (online) http://www. nationmaster.com/country-info/stats/Health/Physicians/ Per-1,000-people.
2. *Forbes.* 2015. (online) http://www.forbes.com/sites/ mikepatton/2015/06/29/u-s-health-care-costs-rise-faster- than-inflation/#1d0f02f26ad2.
3. The Henry J. Kaiser Family Foundation. 2016. (online) http:// kff.org/other/state-indicator/total-active-physicians/? currentTimeframe=0.
4. Rosenthal MB, Zaslavsky A, Newhouse JP. The geographic distribution of physicians revisited. *Health Serv Res.* 2005;*40*:1931–1952.
5. The Henry J. Kaiser Family Foundation. 2016. (online) http://kff.org/other/state-indicator/ total-registered-nurses/?currentTimeframe=0.
6. The Association of Schools of Allied Health Professions (ASAHP). (online) http://www.asahp.org/wp-content/ uploads/2014/08/Health-Professions-Facts.pdf.
7. U.S. Department of Labor, Bureau of Labor Statistics. 2014–2024 projections. (online) https://www.bls.gov/emp/ ep_table_103.htm.

CHAPTER 2

From Cavemen Until Yesterday: An Overview of the Traditional American Healthcare System

To successfully move forward in today's tumultuous healthcare world, therapists, nurses, pharmacists, technicians, other allied health professionals, physicians, and patients will greatly benefit by first looking back. A handful of critical concepts lie at the foundation of all healthcare delivery systems, including the US healthcare system. Appreciating why and how these concepts have changed over time, most dramatically through the recent US healthcare reform movement (which has already been followed by early attempts at reform in numerous other countries[1]), will empower you not only to survive but to truly excel as a healthcare professional. It does not take an advanced degree in healthcare policy or economics to understand how our concept of healthcare has operated for centuries and then why and how reform has become so major a movement. There are a few basic and straightforward concepts that can be easily understood and serve as a foundation on which to build your knowledge of the current evolving healthcare environment.

Appreciating why and how the healthcare system's foundational concepts have changed over time will empower you not only to survive but to truly excel as a healthcare professional.

Broken down into its major elements, all healthcare systems (at the highest level) comprise three significant components:

1. The definition and responsibilities of THE PROVIDER
2. THE COIN OF THE REALM; that is, how the provider is paid (reimbursed)
3. WHAT THE PROVIDER NEEDS to succeed professionally

In this chapter, we will explore these three concepts that lie at the foundation of the US healthcare system as they have existed and functioned throughout the traditional pre-reform healthcare era. Then in subsequent chapters, we will discuss the driving forces of reform and how reform changes and seeks to change THE PROVIDER, THE COIN OF THE REALM, and WHAT THE PROVIDER NEEDS.

For the vast majority of US history, these three foundational healthcare characteristics of US healthcare remained relatively static. Sure, there were minor changes and new forces (as we will touch on briefly in a moment), but viewed from a distance, until recently, US society's concept and beliefs about health and healthcare were stable through time. It is only recently that seismic changes to our basic beliefs about health and healthcare have surfaced, and even currently, we've just dipped our toe into the pool. But again, to understand the world in which you are and will provide patient care, we must first appreciate from where healthcare came.

So, let's move forward by first looking back . . .

The Definition and Responsibilities of

The Provider

Boy, was it great being a doctor! The definition of THE PROVIDER was "The Doctor," and the definition of "The Doctor" was THE PROVIDER. Singular. *The Doctor alone as Provider.* Physicians routinely ranked among the most trusted professions in general surveys of the citizenry.[2] Every mother's dream was that her child would grow up to become a physician (or at worst, grow up to marry a physician). Doctors were seen as honest and ethical.[3] Doctors could do no wrong. Doctors were all-knowing, having learned all the answers in medical school, internship, residency, and through practice. They were not to be questioned. And for the population, this vision was accompanied by overwhelming relief. Relief that when a loved one was injured or fell ill, the brightest medical mind was always available. The doctor would "know what to do," understand the ways of the body, and always deliver the highest quality care (Fig. 2.1).

In all healthcare decisions, *The Doctor was God*. With rare exception, patients did whatever their physicians recommended. Family members rarely questioned the physician's care plan, nor the outcome of the care. The same held true for other caregivers. Nurses followed doctors' orders without question. Pharmacists and technicians filled physician-written prescriptions without hesitation. Dieticians never challenged the doctor's nutritional plans (or lack thereof). Physical and occupational therapists, respiratory therapists, medical assistants . . . all fell in line

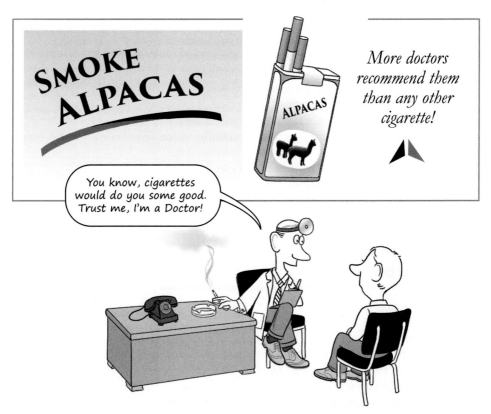

FIGURE 2.1 It seems ironic looking back on advertisements for cigarettes and other products now known to be unhealthy, but physicians were well respected and thoroughly trusted, making them highly coveted spokesmen.

behind the all-knowing physician. Thus not only did the general population view nurses and allied health professionals as standing far below The Doctor on the caregiver ladder, many allied health professionals and nurses viewed themselves similarly as "Caregivers" (yes) but not as "Providers." They were (in fact, still often are) lumped together under the condescending, nondescript label, *"Physician Extenders."* If this nomenclature does not clearly indicate who stood alone at the center of the healthcare world, then I don't know what does.

> In all healthcare decisions, *The Doctor was God.*

In this traditional healthcare model, the physician was responsible for, well, *everything* related to patient care, including numerous areas where other healthcare professionals were eminently more knowledgeable and experienced (and, therefore, able to provide better patient care recommendations, had they been asked more than just occasionally). I remember well practicing as a surgeon for years in this environment. Medications? All up to me, every single one (and with the significant comorbidities found in hospitalized patients, it is not uncommon to need orders for more than a dozen for many individual patients). Physical limitations and activities? Up to me. Diet? Me. Respiratory care? Me again. *Everything was up to me.* Back then (and now, in many care facilities and settings), those of us intelligent enough (or scared enough) to realize that other providers were better educated in these specialized fields would routinely ask for targeted professional guidance. Still, in the vast majority of cases, patient care was a far cry from "collaborative," "interprofessional," or "team driven."

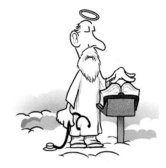

Now, I recognize that the picture I am painting is far too black and white. Certainly "physician extenders" would on occasion question or even push back on portions of a physician's care plan. But for the most part, the doctor was the pilot (and copilot and navigator), and all other caregivers were stewardesses and stewards. And the patient was simply the passive, sleeping passenger in seat 31C.

> In the vast majority of cases, patient care was a far cry from "collaborative," "interprofessional," or "team driven."

Thus, until healthcare reform, the definition and responsibilities of THE PROVIDER followed a simple, ubiquitous equation:

The Provider ⟷ The Doctor

◉ PEARL

In the traditional US system, "The Doctor" is seen as THE PROVIDER, while other caregivers primarily focus on fulfilling the "doctor's orders," and patients routinely play a passive role in their own health and healthcare decisions.

The Coin of the Realm: How The Provider Was Paid

While we are discussing three critical concepts that lay at the heart of all healthcare systems, this feature *(How The Provider Was Paid)* drives the other two. That is, The Coin of the Realm *is the engine of healthcare* and the driver of healthcare reform compliance.

Classic Westerns may exaggerate the financial model of traditional US healthcare, but they are basically accurate.

"Somebody git the doc! A man's been shot!"

Old Doc Barkley races into town on his horse. Carrying his little black bag in one hand, he plows through the double swinging doors of the saloon. Lying prostrate on the billiards table is his patient, blood from the revolver wound in his shoulder darkening the worn, green felt.

Doc Barkley rips open the man's shirt front and back and examines the wounds.

"Yer lucky," he says to the moaning cowboy. "She went clean through."

Then the old doctor proceeds to apply antiseptics, a poultice, and a bandage to both the bullet entrance and exit wounds. With the help of the patient's partners, they sit the injured cowboy up.

"Thanks, Doc," the injured man says. Then, turning to his compadre, he instructs, "Rusty, grab a silver piece out o' my pocket and give it to the Doc."

Rusty complies, fetching a tarnished silver coin from the wounded man's shirt pocket, just below the bloody dressing. He hands it to Doc Barkley.

The doctor pockets the coin and nods at the men.

"If either wound starts to weep or smell, you come 'round and see me."

The patient nods, and old Doc Barkley saunters out of the saloon, the swinging doors marking his exit.

Prior to the recent healthcare reform movement, this is how The Provider was paid. This, the traditional US **healthcare reimbursement model**, is known as **"fee for service."** And these three words by themselves explain the massive machine that is healthcare economics: *providers were paid for providing services.*

THE COIN OF THE REALM is the engine of healthcare and the driver of healthcare reform compliance.

Makes sense, right? After all, when you bring your car to the mechanic to get it repaired, you pay for the service (and any parts). When you take your family out to dinner, you pay for the service (and the food). In fact, our entire US economy is designed to pay for services (and goods). So the fee-for-service provider payment model that drives our traditional US healthcare model is simply another example of "The American Way," right?

Wrong.

Let's dig a little deeper.

If a day after you pick up your car from the repair shop it begins again to make that awful clanking sound, you immediately take it back to the mechanic. If your waiter brings you an overcooked steak, you send it back. And your car is serviced again, and you're brought a properly cooked steak. *Until it's done right. All without any additional payment.* In other words, yes, the US system is predicated upon paying for a service or product *with the expectation that the purchased service or product will be of acceptable quality.* In some cases, the quality of the outcome is clearly stated (a guarantee or warrantee). In other economic sectors, common sense rules the day (as in the restaurant business). But regardless of whether clearly stated, legislated, or uniformly understood, the American Way includes an explicit understanding (unless otherwise clearly stated) that *there is a direct relationship between payment and the quality* of the purchased service or goods.

Not so in the healthcare fee-for-service model. In this bizarre economic world, *there is no meaningful relationship between the payment to the service provider and the quality of the outcome experienced by the consumer.* (Although the explosion in medical lawsuits addresses some poor-quality care, clinical outcomes and provider reimbursement have overall remained unlinked.) In fact, in the fee-for-service reimbursement model, *payment and quality are perversely inversely related.* Take this example:

I attempt to perform a challenging cancer operation for which I am not adequately trained or experienced (and believe me, sadly, this is not an uncommon occurrence within hospitals all over the country and the world). As a result, my female patient suffers a serious complication during surgery, a complication that would have been avoided had the operation been performed by a more experienced cancer surgeon. This **preventable medical error** requires my injured-and-now-very-ill patient to be cared for in the intensive care unit (ICU). Had the avoidable complication actually been avoided, she would not have needed this complex, laborious, expensive ICU care. In fact, my patient would have stayed less than a week on the surgical ward before being discharged home.

If I had not made an avoidable mistake. If my patient had not suffered a preventable medical error.

Now, back to my "little mishap" . . . during my patient's unanticipated ICU stay, a nurse caring for her inadvertently administered triple the dosage of a powerful antibiotic medication, which temporarily damaged my patient's kidneys. (The nurse, overwhelmed by the complexity of her two very sick ICU patients, made a preventable medical error.) Until my patient's kidneys could recover, she had to undergo regular hemodialysis (an exhausting and costly mechanical waste-filtering process that mimics normal kidney function) to survive the nurse's avoidable mistake (which itself was set up by my preventable medical error).

Unfortunately, the (avoidable) surgical complication didn't heal on its own, and I had to perform a second surgical procedure to repair the (preventable) damage that occurred (I caused) during the original operation.

Following this second (avoidable) operation, my patient remained on (preventable) hemodialysis in the ICU for 2 more weeks, as her (avoidably damaged) kidneys slowly recovered. Then, at last, my patient was stable enough to move from the ICU to the surgical ward (where she would have recovered and from where she would already have been discharged weeks ago, had the first procedure gone as it should have or had she received the correct medication dose in the ICU). My patient's kidneys recovered, and 2 weeks later she is finally discharged from the hospital to a rehabilitation facility (which would not have been necessary if she had not been the victim of two preventable medical errors). Six weeks later, my patient is finally discharged home from the rehabilitation facility (2 months later than she would have returned to her home and her family had the quality of her surgical and ICU care been appropriate).

We can all agree that from the patient's perspective (and that of her family and friends, as well as her employer, her insurance provider, and the taxpayers [if her care was government subsidized]), the quality of her care was extremely poor. Worse than picking up your car from the mechanic only to find that the car still makes that horrible, clanking sound. But unlike the mechanic at the repair shop, here's where the healthcare fee-for-service business model wildly diverges[4,5] from the rest of our economic model: *the doctor* (who makes an avoidable mistake) *and the nurse or health professional* (who makes an avoidable mistake) *and the hospital* (which credentials and/or employs the doctor, nurse, and allied health professionals who make avoidable mistakes) *routinely all get paid to care for and treat the preventable injuries that they caused!*

> In the fee-for-service reimbursement model, payment and quality are perversely inversely related.

In this example, I made an avoidable mistake in the operating room (obviously impossible!). The ICU nurse made an avoidable medication dosing error which badly damaged my patient's kidneys, sending her to dialysis and requiring a 2-week stay in the ICU. And because of the nurse's employment and my employment and/or surgical privileging, the hospital also bears some culpability. And yet, *we all got paid!* Not only for the first operation, but *also for the second (avoidable) operation. And for the entire (avoidable) ICU stay. And for the weeks of (avoidable) hemodialysis. And for the (avoidable) prolonged surgical ward care. And for a 6-week (avoidable) stay in the rehabilitation facility.*

> In the Bizarro World of healthcare fee-for-service economics, there is no meaningful relationship between the payment to the service provider and the quality of the outcome experienced by the consumer.

In other words, if the auto repair industry mimicked healthcare, you would not only have to pay the mechanic for finally actually repairing your car, *you would also have to pay for the parts and labor billed the first time, when he failed to fix your car.* Your steak is overcooked? No problem, provided that you not only pay for the second, correctly cooked steak *but for the first overcooked slab as well* (and tip your waiter double).

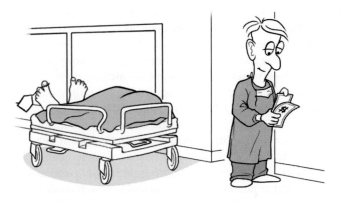

A couple of important points here. First of all, understanding the fee-for-service model can clearly lead to the assumption that doctors, hospital staff, and hospitals don't mind delivering poor-quality care or even *seek to do so for financial gain.* After all, making mistakes means more money for all of us!

Nothing could be further from the truth. Healthcare is a calling, not a cash cow. Yes, nurses and health providers (and physicians) make very solid livings: the median salary for a registered nurse in the United States in 2015 was $67,490[6] and for a physical therapist was $84,020.[7] But consider that the 4 years required to become a registered nurse can cost between $55,000 and $100,000,[8] and a doctorate—the more favored degree—in physical therapy can cost between $35,000 and $75,000.[9] Allied health professionals, nurses, physicians, and other care providers spend years paying for educations and then work long hours because—as corny as it sounds—we are dedicated to helping our patients. But despite our best efforts and plans, the practice of medicine is still far from an "exact science." It is heavily dependent on the judgment and skills of individual people and, therefore, highly prone to preventable errors and avoidable mistakes that harm, even kill, patients.

So how has quality care delivery been championed? What "checks and balances" have been put in place within our traditional fee-for-service system to ensure some expectation of quality care and/or some reasonable corrective processes to ensure the avoidance of repeated preventable mistakes?

> Despite our best efforts and plans, the practice of medicine is still far from an "exact science." It is heavily dependent on the judgment and skills of individual people and, therefore, highly prone to preventable errors and avoidable mistakes that harm, even kill, patients.

◉ PEARL

The traditional US healthcare system (which still predominates currently in many US care settings) is based on the *fee-for-service* model, in which provider reimbursement is disconnected from the quality of care delivered and resultant patient outcomes.

In actuality, few if any meaningful quality-enabling processes have been universally incorporated into our healthcare system prior to the recent reform efforts. That said, there has been one major and truly impactful process that has arisen over the past several decades, an action aimed much more at penalizing than at preventing poor care and suboptimal patient outcomes: ***malpractice litigation.*** Now, had malpractice litigation been developed, implemented, and modified in a standardized and thoughtful manner, had it been envisioned to *drive improvement in care quality* through the avoidance of preventable mistakes, it is likely that medical malpractice litigation might actually have benefited our society. And although it is rare that a lawsuit sustainably elevates the quality of care delivery on a large scale, financially punishing providers and provider institutions for the delivery of truly suboptimal care is arguably a very reasonable and critical societal action. Unfortunately, many malpractice lawsuits are driven by another goal: making money. This is not always true for the plaintiffs, many of whom are truly primarily seeking to "make sure that what happened to our loved one never happens to any other patient again." However, malpractice has been hijacked by numerous "ambulance chasing" attorneys and "injured" patients who are willing to abandon their principles and ethics in search of the almighty dollar. Thus was the birth of the ***frivolous malpractice lawsuit.*** A *2006 New England Journal of Medicine* study determined that "For 3% of the [filed medical negligence] claims, there were no verifiable medical injuries, and 37% did not involve errors."[10] And get this: 28% of these frivolous claims resulted in some form of payment.

As the medical malpractice industry cranked up at warp speed, it was minimally regulated in any meaningful way (cynically argued as the result of the majority of legislators being lawyers). Soon, there was a predictable explosion in frivolous lawsuits. And I mean *truly frivolous*. I remember the first time I was named in a medical malpractice suit . . .

I was so excited! After 4 years of medical school, followed by 8 grueling years of surgical training, I had been hired by a premier Southern California surgical group as only the sixth (and youngest) member of the practice. In the first few months, they never left me alone in the operating room, even if I knew how to do a surgical procedure that was new or unfamiliar to them. They did this to protect my initial reputation in the referring medical community, feeling that should anything ever go wrong during my first months, their presence would indicate that I, the new junior surgeon, was not at fault.

I never would have imagined that the first lawsuit in which I was named would occur so early into my surgical career. Let alone *following an operation and hospital recovery that went without a hitch.* I had not even been the primary surgeon, instead assisting my senior partner, who was a talented and experienced operator. He had flawlessly removed a short segment of diseased intestine. Our female patient had experienced an uneventful recovery, returning home from the surgical ward only 5 days following her operation.

And yet some 6 months later, both my senior partner and I (along with the hospital) were named as defendants in a medical malpractice suit, accused of providing "negligent medical care."

I would not wish being named a defendant in a lawsuit on my worst enemy (OK . . . maybe on my *worst* enemy). I couldn't sleep. I couldn't eat. I was constantly depressed. Anyone who has ever been so named knows that endless, painful, grinding in the pit of your stomach that goes on day and night.

My senior partner (who had served as primary surgeon) had been sued several times previously. More than 15% of general surgeons, and an even higher proportion of some surgical specialists, are sued *annually.*[11] With this legal action, as with each of its predecessors, my senior partner also could not sleep or eat and wandered around in a state of disillusionment.

Then an even more inexplicable thing occurred: *the patient who was suing us showed up at our office for her scheduled 6-month follow-up visit.* She was not angry when, through our receptionist, we refused to see her. This was a permissible refusal, given that this visit was not an emergency visit (since the lawsuit was filed, we had provided her with a list of competent, local physicians who could assume her care) and also *given that she was suing us for malpractice.* However, she was very upset, even crying that we were her doctors, and we were the best, and she needed us to care for her.

My senior partner, ever the professional, chose to speak with the woman in hopes of calming her and allowing her to understand why we could no longer care for her. He signaled silently for me to follow.

"Hello, Ms. Babcock [not her real name]," he said stoically but without any apparent hostility. "I'm sorry, but given that you're suing me, my colleague here, Dr. Edelstein, and our hospital, our attorneys have advised us not to communicate with you in any way or provide care for you unless it is an emergency."

"But . . ." she stammered, tears literally overflowing her eyes, *"you take such good care of me!"*

My senior partner remained calm. "Thank you. Then, may I ask, *why are you suing us?*"

With no hint of embarrassment and absolute confidence in her answer, she replied. "My attorney said that if I sue you and the hospital, the hospital will drop all of my medical charges rather than go to court. And he promised me, *he promised me,* that a suit wouldn't hurt you, because you have malpractice insurance."

My senior partner reflected for a moment. Then he gently reached for her hand, which she took gratefully. "Well, I'm afraid that's far from the truth. In fact, your lawsuit hurts me and Dr. Edelstein, here, in two significant ways. First, it costs us money for our attorneys to review your lawsuit, because ultimately our insurance premiums rise. And if we end up going to court, it costs us a lot more in time away from our practice, win or lose. And if we do lose, or even if we settle without going to court, it raises our insurance costs. Just like if you're in a car accident, your insurance premiums can go up, right?"

His noncondescending tone and gentle manner encouraged her to nod in the affirmative.

"And I'm afraid that the other damage caused by your lawsuit is even worse. Dr. Edelstein and I have worked very hard for years. We work at night and on weekends because we've committed ourselves to caring for surgical patients like you. And *a lawsuit damages our reputation in the community.* Because, Ms. Babcock, no one will assume that you're suing us to avoid having to pay your hospital bill."

He said this without a hint of criticism, his voice entirely void of negative judgment.

"No," he continued. "Everyone will assume that I did something wrong in your care. That I made an inexcusable mistake during your operation. That I did something I should have known not to do when I cared for you."

He stopped speaking. She looked at him with an expression of bewilderment and shame. He gently swayed her hand and concluded.

"Your lawsuit threatens *my reputation* as well as my livelihood."

They spoke further for several minutes as my mind tried to organize something logical out of all that I had heard. She had experienced no medical or surgical complications. She had not one single complaint about the care she had received. *She still desperately wanted my partner to care for her!* She had simply believed, based on misleading information and encouragement provided by her attorney, that by suing her doctors and the hospital, she could avoid having to pay her insurance deductible, assured (again by her lawyer) that the suit would carry no negative consequences for her wonderful surgeon.

Within a day of this bizarre encounter, Ms. Babcock's attorney notified our attorneys that our names had been removed from the suit. The hospital now remained the sole defendant. And although the nurses, allied health professionals, administrators, and other hospital staff had in actuality taken excellent and appropriate care of Ms. Babcock, in the end her attorney was right about one thing: rather than pay to fight the clearly frivolous lawsuit, the hospital simply retracted her bill and ate the costs.

So, Ms. Babcock won. And Ms. Babcock's unethical attorney won. Nor is money the only thing that my hospital lost in giving in to Ms. Babcock's baseless lawsuit. Just as my senior partner explained, *reputations are damaged by lawsuits.* Simply the perception that the hospital (via its nurses, allied health professionals, and other staff) made an avoidable mistake in caring for a patient damages the hospital, all who work in the hospital, and the surrounding community. And believe me, having worked in both large and small hospital systems, these "little" reputational hits add up.

And of course in absorbing the actual costs of Ms. Babcock's care, the hospital lost money. Albeit not a lot of money, but *their honestly earned money.* And ultimately, *every one of us who pays directly and/or indirectly into the US healthcare system loses money in this and similar scams.* The endless little financial hits that our healthcare system undeservedly takes at the urging of unprincipled lawyers and unethical patients are akin to shoplifting. People often wonder why the big, billion-dollar stores give a hoot about the woman who pockets cheap lipstick without paying. Or the man who slips a magazine into the folds of his coat. After all, these are just infinitesimal financial losses . . .

Every one of us who pays directly and/or indirectly into the US healthcare system loses money through frivolous malpractice lawsuits.

In 2015, US commercial stores lost more than $32,000,000,000 (that's 32 *billion*) to shoplifters.[12] That is the cumulative effect of these little piecemeal thefts. And just who do you think pays for that whopping rip-off? *You do. I do. We all do.* Through higher store prices (come on . . . you don't honestly believe that the stores simply suck up the losses rather than pass them on to the consumer). It's the same in healthcare. Ever wonder why the insurance premium deduction from your monthly paycheck is so high (check it!) even though you and your family are healthy? I'm generalizing, of course, as the calculation of the cost of everything from an in-hospital pain pill to insurance coverage is far more complicated. But so is the retail sales business. Shoplifting is just one component that is factored into the costs of goods offered across the shelves of US retail stores. And just as thousands of tiny, inexpensive individual items slipped silently into the clothes of shoplifters raise store prices, frivolous lawsuits significantly impact the cost of healthcare for us all.

Although the costs of frivolous malpractice lawsuits certainly contribute, the main fuel behind the United State's skyrocketing healthcare costs has been the healthcare community's response to the constant threat of medical negligence claims: the development and practice of **"defensive medicine."** When care providers practice out of fear of "missing something," even something that would *not be reasonably (statistically) be expected or anticipated*, fear that future "experts" may retrospectively scrutinize every single one of their past care actions (with the benefit of hindsight), then those providers will no longer practice **patient-centered care;** we are practicing *attorney-centered care.* Surveys of US physicians acknowledge this terrible shift in the focus of care from patient to attorney: "75 percent of doctors say that they order more tests, procedures and medicines than are medically necessary in an attempt to avoid lawsuits."[13]

The practice of defensive medicine has had a devastating effect on US healthcare. The ordering of tests, procedures, and medications that are clinically and statistically of no benefit to patients not only needlessly drives up healthcare costs, but also exposes patients to the risks associated with those unnecessary diagnostic tests and treatments. In addition, defensive medicine wastes valuable resources, delaying care for patients who truly need certain tests, therapies, and provider attention. Here is a common, real-world example:

> Your 8-year-old son complains of some pain around his belly button soon after you pick him up from school. You take his temperature, and it is a little high. He turns down brownies and milk, unheard of in your experience . . . your little man is really feeling lousy.
>
> By dinner time, he's lying in bed, refusing dinner, and complaining that the pain's now far worse. He's holding his stomach just above his right groin. And now he's a little nauseated.
>
> Time to head to the ER.
>
> The ER nurse confirms that your son has a low-grade fever. A phlebotomist gently draws his blood, and your boy provides a urine sample. The ER doc, a friendly sort, examines him gently. Still, your son almost comes off the table when the physician pushes lightly on his belly just above the right groin.
>
> "The blood test and your son's exam tell us that he has appendicitis."
>
> "Appendicitis?" you say more than ask, nodding. "So he needs to have his appendix taken out?"
>
> The ER doc nods. "I'll call the surgeon to come see you." Then he pauses momentarily before adding, "But first we'll get an ultrasound, just to be sure."
>
> Although he's been given some pain medication, your son is still very uncomfortable. And you've heard about an appendix that "burst" because it wasn't promptly taken out. So you're a bit worried about the 45-minute wait until a very pleasant transportation technician comes to take your son for an ultrasound. The sonographer is compassionate and gentle, but the study still causes your son to flinch and moan as the probe is pushed down over his inflamed appendix.
>
> Twenty minutes after your son returns, the ER doc returns. "Yep, the ultrasound shows that it's likely appendicitis."
>
> *"Likely?"* You repeat, the hesitation obvious in your voice.
>
> "Well . . . yes," the ER physician answers, realizing that with that one simple word, "likely," he has opened a Pandora's box. "I mean, just to be sure, we *could* do a CAT scan . . ."

Your miserable son now waits an hour-and-a-half before being wheeled off for a CAT scan. He's back in the ER 2 hours after the completion of his initial ultrasound study, which showed appendicitis, itself performed almost an hour after the ER doctor's clear diagnosis was . . . appendicitis.

Thirty minutes later, the surgeon arrives in the ER A serious, gray-haired man wearing green scrubs, he first examines your son's ER chart and then examines your son.

"Your son has appendicitis. We'll need to take it out right away."

"Right away" is obviously a relative term in this all-too-common scenario.

Ask any experienced surgeon (or ER physician, or even radiologist): the diagnosis of acute appendicitis in an 8-year-old boy with the classic symptoms (vague pain around the belly button that moves down and to the right, low-grade fever, loss of appetite, mild nausea) and the classic signs (focal tenderness over the inflamed appendix, low-grade temperature elevation, slightly elevated white blood cell count) does not require any radiologic studies. The boy could immediately be taken to the operating room for removal of his inflamed appendix. That said, even in the absence of malpractice litigation, most doctors nowadays would accept the minimal delay and order a quick ultrasound study. Ultrasound is safe and cost effective. Most importantly, in classically presenting cases, an ultrasound diagnosis of an acutely inflamed appendix is highly accurate.[14]

In such clear-cut situations (a male child with a classic history, physical exam, lab results, and ultrasound findings), the addition of a diagnostic abdominal-pelvic CAT scan:

- Offers no meaningful clinical benefit to the patient
- Requires that the patient experience pain and other symptoms for longer (often hours more)
- Adds the minor risk of the appendix perforating during the unnecessary delay
- Wastes money (emergency, in-hospital CAT scans cost thousands of dollars)
- Wastes the time of the ER nurse, transportation tech, CAT scan tech, and others (these staff members are valuable resources)
- Requires patients who truly need an emergency CAT scan to wait

And yet every day across the United States (and much of the world), little boys with the classic signs and symptoms and findings of acute appendicitis are subjected to unnecessary CAT scans that tell their doctors what they already know: the little boys have acute appendicitis.

This is defensive medicine. Done on the one-in-a-million chance that the boy's classic signs and symptoms, classic blood tests, classic ultrasound are all wrong and that the CAT scan will somehow find what everything has missed (the true cause of the child's illness). But even if the patient has a rare condition that is not diagnosed prior to surgery, here is what happens: the child undergoes a safe, simple, short operation that is of little true risk; upon finding a "normal" appendix, the surgeon thoroughly examines the patient's entire abdomen and pelvis to identify (and if appropriate, surgically address) the actual cause of the patient's illness.

So why do the unnecessary and wasteful CAT scan? Because if this little boy is that one-in-a-million, and if somehow the safe, simple, short operation still fails to identify the real problem, and if that undiscovered real problem later injures that little boy, *the ER doctor, the surgeon, the radiologist, and the hospital (which employs the ER and OR nurses and allied health professionals) will be sued.*

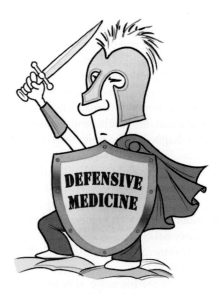

Care decisions should be driven by knowledge, not by malpractice attorneys and statistical rarities. That is, *healthcare should be based on scientific evidence, not fear.*

And it is no exaggeration that, although rare, the performance of unnecessary tests and procedures (defensive medicine) can actually *place patients at significant risk.* Here is another example from my clinical past.

I first met Jerry when I was called by his panicking medical resident.

"Can you come right away?" The young physician's voice was filled with fear. "I think he's bleeding to death!"

He was right. Jerry was bleeding to death.

In his mid-40s, Jerry had for the past several months been experiencing a dull, aching pain "deep in his stomach." As part of his outpatient evaluation, his physician had ordered a CAT scan of his abdomen— an appropriate test, given that Jerry's simpler initial diagnostic tests had failed to shed any light on the source of his pain. The CAT scan also detected nothing to explain Jerry's dull pain. What it *had* found, *incidentally,* was a tiny, circular lesion (abnormality) in Jerry's liver. The experienced radiologist diagnosed this as a benign lesion of no clinical significance to the patient and was confident that this small lesion was absolutely not the source of Jerry's pain. The liver finding was simply an "incidentaloma," the term used in healthcare to refer to the common identification of unexpected findings on imaging studies and other tests.

Such incidentalomas are extremely common findings on CAT scans, often identified in the liver, kidneys, and even adrenal glands in the radiographic search for something else. If the radiologist has any clinical concerns about an incidentaloma, he or she recommends additional safe imaging studies to better diagnose the finding. Because the vast majority of these little radiologic surprises are benign (not cancer, not infections, not dangerous), clinical experience and medical evidence tells us that they should be left alone, as if never discovered, and never to be of any import to those who unknowingly harbor them. The uncommon incidentaloma that is mildly concerning (as a potentially dangerous lesion) is easily reevaluated several months later (through a follow-up CAT scan or other imaging study). If it has changed or grown in a seemingly threatening way, treatment is considered. Very rarely, an incidentaloma concerns the radiologist enough that invasive evaluation is recommended, usually in the form of a biopsy.

Jerry's "incidental finding" posed no diagnostic challenge for the radiologist. It was classic for a common, benign liver growth of no consequence. The recommendation was to simply ignore it, or if Jerry's physician had any concerns, that the incidentaloma be reevaluated for change via a CAT scan in 6 months.

Enter attorney-centric, defensive medical care . . .

What if the radiologist was wrong? What if that bump in Jerry's liver (that no one would even have ever known about had Jerry not undergone a CAT scan looking for something else) was not what the *(experienced, confident)* radiologist said it was? What if Jerry had won the Losers' Lotto and that little nodule in his liver was that one-in-a-million, life-threatening tumor?

Such thinking, as was demonstrated by Jerry's physicians, *was not based on doing what was best for Jerry,* was not guided by credible medical evidence and experience. It was classic defensive medicine, based on the fear that someday, some "expert" will support an attorney in claiming that to leave Jerry's liver "condition" undiagnosed was "malpractice."

And so, ignoring not only the radiologist's diagnosis and experienced recommendation, but also denying all clinical evidence and experience, Jerry's physicians arranged for Jerry to undergo a biopsy of his liver incidentaloma. Under the guidance of another CAT scan, the interventional radiologist passed a long needle through the skin of Jerry's belly and deep into Jerry's liver, aiming to retrieve a tiny portion of the tiny growth to prove (as the radiologist was certain of) that it posed no danger to Jerry.

Not surprisingly (given that the liver is basically a massive sponge filled with blood), Jerry's liver bled. *Like the proverbial stuck pig.* Jerry required multiple blood transfusions (which carry complication risks, infectious risks, waste a valuable limited resource, and cost money), but still his physicians could not keep up with his massive bleeding.

Enter me and my surgical team. Yep, we had to rush Jerry to the operating room, where he underwent a major operation to save his life by stopping the massive bleeding from the needle that had been unnecessarily driven through his liver to take a sample of an incidentaloma which, days later, was confirmed to be entirely benign, exactly as the radiologist had initially said.

Jerry survived his unnecessary biopsy. After many days in the ICU, a couple more weeks in the hospital, and then months off work, he returned to his normal life.

And his dull, abdominal pain continued, never diagnosed.

Oh yeah. The second CAT scan, the needle biopsy, all that blood, the operation, the ICU, the weeks in the hospital? All that completely unnecessary, 100% avoidable care?

All paid for.

CAT scans. Blood tests. Urine studies. Daily chest x-rays. Biopsies (which carry real risk). Antibiotics. MRIs. Blood transfusions. It is estimated that in 2009, $750 billion (approximately 30% of all medical costs)[15,16] was spent unnecessarily, and there is no reason to believe that trend has declined. That translates into thousands (more likely tens of thousands) of unnecessary medical diagnostic tests and procedures performed across this country every single day. Tests and procedures that routinely delay and/or confuse the appropriate diagnosis and/or patient treatment processes. Tests and procedures that waste valuable resources. Tests and procedures that waste billions of dollars. Tests and procedures that can even place patients at risk.

And *tests and procedures that the evidence-based literature shows us, and healthcare providers often recognize, offer no meaningful benefit to our patients.*

Thousands of unnecessary medical diagnostic tests and procedures are performed across this country every single day . . . tests and procedures that the evidence-based literature shows us, and healthcare providers often recognize, offer no meaningful benefit to our patients.

Unfortunately, the practice of defensive medicine and the filing of frivolous lawsuits still thrive despite the current world of healthcare reform. Before the passage of the ACA, respected healthcare economists and commentators openly anticipated that in the absence of *meaningful, federally legislated malpractice litigation reform* **(tort reform),** mandated healthcare reform would fall short of its potential (still, the ACA contained no tort reform).[17,18] And the call for tort reform currently continues.[19–22] It is true that many states have attempted differing forms of tort reform (even prior to the passage of the ACA in 2010); however, with few exceptions, these varying state approaches have failed to consistently demonstrate any impact on the on the quality of US healthcare.[23]

The skyrocketing cost of US healthcare is driven in part by that outrageously expensive, unnecessary byproduct of the threat of malpractice litigation: the universal practice of defensive medicine.

The reality is that even if representatives of both the legal sector and healthcare were open to meaningful discussion on the topic of tort reform (which itself would be an achievement), the issue itself is far from black and white. Ask an attorney, and you'll likely hear them defend the need to hold healthcare providers accountable for medical negligence (an argument that even the most defensive caregiver would likely admit is reasonable). Ask a provider and you'll likely hear about clearly frivolous lawsuits that drive up healthcare costs and insurance premiums and damage reputations (an argument with which any ethical attorney would agree). But many malpractice lawsuits fall somewhere in between these two, clear-cut extremes. What exactly defines "negligent care?" How much money should a patient receive for an outcome that many would see as insignificant? What's the price of an avoidable death? And was it truly avoidable or was the patient just that ill?

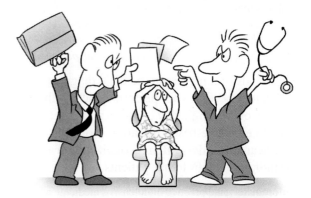

Tort reform will not be easy. But *it is necessary* if we are to reduce the enormous waste (both financial and otherwise) resulting from the practice of defensive medicine.

So in the end, THE COIN OF THE REALM in the fee-for-service world is just that: a coin. *Money.* With no relationship to outcomes or quality of care. And countered by a tremendously damaging medical malpractice environment in which, although potentially helping those truly injured through negligent care, we all end up paying unimaginable amounts of money to support the practice of defensive medicine and the settling of frivolous lawsuits.

⊙ **PEARL**

The explosion in medical malpractice litigation has led to the extremely costly practice (in terms of money and many nonfinancial outcomes) of *defensive medicine,* which currently persists, with the absence of universal, meaningful *tort reform.*

In the end, THE COIN OF THE REALM in the fee-for-service world is just that: a coin. Money. With no relationship to outcomes or quality of care.

But lawsuits aside (both legitimate and frivolous), *our traditional fee-for-service healthcare system is defined by a critical disconnection between the outcomes experienced by the patient and the compensation realized by the provider.* And it has been this model of healthcare that Americans (and many other nations around the globe) have adopted and accepted for ages. But now *it is this fee-for-service healthcare system that has driven the United States (and many of those other nations around the globe) to horrifically poor health among their populations and costs of care that are pushing towards financial disaster.*

What THE PROVIDER Needs

So for centuries, things have been pretty simple. "Provider" meant "Doctor," and physicians were clearly the Gods of All Healthcare Decisions. Fee for service meant that providers could practice without realizing financial risk related to the quality of the care they delivered. The physician was rarely if ever questioned and made all care-related decisions, safe in the knowledge that the fee-for-service model meant payment without regard to patient outcome. Providers and provider institutions soon learned to limit malpractice litigation risk though the routine overprescribing of unnecessary, costly, and occasionally risky tests and procedures; that is, by practicing defensive medicine. Although for the most part, patients, nurses, therapists, and other allied health professionals moved silently and unnoticed through the health and healthcare world, simply "following the doctor's orders."

Yep, *it was a great time to be a doctor!*

So what did THE PROVIDER (The Doctor) need in serving as undisputed, unaccountable healthcare leader? Not much, really. All a provider needed to be considered a credible practitioner of medicine, and thus to receive payment for care, was a medical degree in a black frame hanging crookedly on his or her office wall. As for keeping current with credible, evidence-based information, the need to keep abreast of the massive quantity of ever-changing scientific guidance directing "the best care," it was entirely up to the individual physician. Doctors could choose to define "keeping current" as they saw fit. And to be fair, most doctors did and do wish to stay up to date with the most recent knowledge regarding the care of their own patients. What that meant for most physicians was office shelves crammed full with textbooks and journals. Now, many doctors religiously read articles that provide current information, striving to deliver the safest, most beneficial care. But you know the old saying: *"The road to Hell . . ."* The reality for most physicians was and is that in our hectic hours filled with emergencies and ever-more crowed waiting rooms, taking time to read last month's journals falls to the bottom of the priority list (especially when up against time with family or even sleep). Furthermore, particularly prior to the recent explosion in mobile technology, the most current knowledge was scripted in ink across the printed pages of books and journals, hidden in distant, dark, offices, far from the exam room and patient bedside where the vast majority of clinical care decisions were made.

All a provider needed to be considered a credible practitioner of medicine, and thus to receive payment for care, was a medical degree in a black frame hanging crookedly on his or her office wall.

Thus, *in real time, physicians relied heavily on their previous training, personal experience, and professional judgment ("gut feeling") in directing patient care.* Fortunately, things have recently (historically speaking) changed dramatically: the availability of current, credible, evidence-based information literally at our fingertips anytime, anywhere, has dramatically eased the ability of all care providers (including patients) in finding scientifically credible care guidance. (That said, source "credibility" and other concerns have been introduced by our newfound technological access to healthcare information, and these must be acknowledged and addressed).

PEARL

Given the fee-for-service structure and the focus on the doctor, physicians relied (and to a large extent still rely) on their own training, personal experiences, and professional judgment in determining care recommendations.

Putting It All Together: The Traditional Healthcare System

So there you have it. The stage is set. You now understand the three critical, foundational themes of the traditional US healthcare system that preceded the recent and ongoing reform revolution and which currently in many areas of the country continue to define US healthcare:

- The Doctor is the sole PROVIDER, and the Doctor is God;
- THE COIN OF THE REALM is money, with the quality of patient care outcomes having little influence on clinical practice;
- THE PROVIDER only needed medical legitimacy (provided via a medical degree) to be considered credible practitioners.

And the reason I have led you through this laborious chapter is so that *you now have a baseline for understanding Act II: Healthcare Reform*. Because with reform, THE COIN OF THE REALM changed dramatically; and this meant that the definition, roles, and responsibilities of THE PROVIDER had to undergo a titanic evolution; and this necessitated a colossal expansion in What THE PROVIDER Needs to succeed in the current healthcare world.

Exciting, yes? Then *read on*!

References

1. Maday M, Drobnick E, McClellan M. *Studying health care reform abroad: lessons in chronic disease management*. Brookings; 2015 [online]. https://www.brookings.edu/blog/health360/2015/07/22/studying-health-care-reform-abroad-lessons-in-chronic-disease-management.
2. Blendon RJ, Benson JM, Hero JO. Public trust in physicians—U.S. medicine in international perspective. *N Engl J Med.* 2014;371:1570–1572.
3. Gallup (online); http://www.gallup.com/poll/1654/honesty-ethics-professions.aspx.
4. Mello MM, Studdert DM, Thomas EJ, Yoon CS, Brennan TA. Who pays for medical errors? An analysis of adverse event costs, the medical liability system, and incentives for patient safety improvement. *J Empirical Legal Stud.* 2007;4:835–860.
5. Luthra S. *A medical mistake happens. Who pays the bill?* The Washington Post; 2015 [online]. https://www.washingtonpost.com/national/health-science/a-medical-mistake-happens-who-pays-the-bill/2015/11/09/9d4f6ee6-78d1-11e5-b9c1-f03c48c96ac2_story.html?utm_term=.f1bfca39e5fa.
6. U.S. News & World Report (online); http://money.usnews.com/careers/best-jobs/registered-nurse/salary.
7. U.S. News & World Report (online); http://money.usnews.com/careers/best-jobs/physical-therapist/salary.
8. RegisteredNurseEducationRequirements.net (online); http://www.registerednurseeducationrequirements.net/Registered-Nurse-Education-Costs.html.
9. CostHelper Education (online); http://education.costhelper.com/physical-therapist-school.html.
10. Studdert DM, Mello MM, Gawande AA, et al. Claims, errors, and compensation payments in medical malpractice litigation. *N Engl J Med.* 2006;354:2024–2033.
11. Jena AB, Seabury S, Lakdawalla D, Chandra A. Malpractice risk according to physician specialty. *N Engl J Med.* 2012;365:629–636.
12. Wahba P. *Shoplifting, worker theft cost retailers $32 billion last year*. Fortune; 2015 [online]. http://fortune.com/2015/06/24/shoplifting-worker-theft-cost-retailers-32-billion-in-2014/?iid=sr-link1.
13. Scherz H, Oliver W. *Defensive medicine: a cure worse than the disease*. Forbes; 2013 [online]. http://www.forbes.com/sites/realspin/2013/08/27/defensive-medicine-a-cure-worse-than-the-disease/#e896398358fe.

14. Lourenco P, Brown J, Leipsic J, Hague C. The current utility of ultrasound in the diagnosis of acute appendicitis. *Clin Imaging.* 2016;40:944–948.

15. Institute of Medicine. *Best care at lower cost: the path to continuously learning health care in America*; 2012 [online]. http://www.nationalacademies.org/hmd/Reports/2012/Best-Care-at-Lower-Cost-The-Path-to-Continuously-Learning-Health-Care-in-America.aspx.

16. Haelle T. *Putting tests to the test: many medical procedures prove unnecessary—and risky.* Scientific American; 2013 [online]. https://www.scientificamerican.com/article/medical-procedures-prove-unnecessary.

17. Benoit S. *Tort reform can lower costs without harming health care. So why isn't it in Obama's plan?* PJ Media; 2009 [online]. https://pjmedia.com/blog/tort-reform-aids-health-lowers-cost-why-isnt-it-in-obamacare.

18. Nix K, Sherwood R. *Big tort means big problems for US health care.* The Daily Signal; 2010 [online]. http://dailysignal.com//2010/02/04/big-tort-means-big-problems-for-us-health-care.

19. Sage WM, Hyman D. Let's make a deal: trading malpractice reform for health reform. *Health Aff.* 2014;33:53–58.

20. Corapi S. *Could malpractice reform save the U.S. health care system?* PBS NewsHour; 2014 [online]. http://www.pbs.org/newshour/rundown/could-malpractice-reform-save-the-us-health-care-system.

21. Stimson CJ, Dmochowski R, Penson DF. Health care reform 2010: a fresh view on tort reform. *J Urol.* 2010;184:1840–1846.

22. Butler PD, Chang B, Britt LD. The affordable care act and academic surgery: expectations and possibilities. *J Am Coll Surg.* 2014;218:1049–1055.

23. Floyd TK. Medical malpractice: trends in litigation. *Gastroenterology.* 2008;7:1822–1825.

CHAPTER 3

A Whole New World: The Forces Behind the Healthcare Reform Revolution

Healthcare reform has been a hot political topic for decades upon decades. So you shouldn't be surprised to learn that the current reform movement is not the first to attempt to broadly change healthcare in this country. However, while piecemeal aspects of previous reform initiatives have survived, today's US healthcare reform revolution truly differs from previous iterations. Healthcare reform today represents the first time that *federal legislation has been passed, fundamentally changing not only how we are to view healthcare, but how we should view health.* (This legislation, the **Affordable Care Act,** or **ACA,** is widely referred to as "**ObamaCare.**") And as we'll discuss, the driving realities and powerful forces that have combined so strongly to push reform that have emboldened political leaders to mandate what is nothing less than an entirely new approach to American healthcare will not easily be ignored or reversed in the future.

> Healthcare reform today represents the first time that *federal legislation has been passed, fundamentally changing not only how we are to view healthcare, but how we should view health.*

This in no way means that healthcare reform in America won't undergo change. Not possible. Reform as currently legislated will surely undergo change. *Radical* change, more likely than not. Even as I pen this chapter, 7 years after the ACA was signed into law, the debate over healthcare reform rages both in the marble hallways of Capitol Hill and along the tree-lined avenues of Main Street, United States. But this is not entirely (or even mainly) due to politics. Healthcare is so complex, so deeply integrated within societies, so large a portion of the American economy, and yet so personal, that it is impossible for any nation to "get it right the first time." Thus, outside of the United States, similar iterative reform processes have already occurred. In Australia, for example, initial attempts at reform focused heavily on increasing the number of Australians enrolled in private health insurance plans and on the introduction of **health information technology (HIT)** solutions into the provider workflow. These initial reform strategies have largely been viewed as having failed,[1,2] requiring modifications to the original federal healthcare reform organizational structure and changes to the initial strategies. The United Kingdom, too, is struggling through attempts to improve the cost-efficiency of their National Health System,[3,4] and both governments have been the target of scathing criticism in the lay press.

Reform as currently legislated will surely undergo change. *Radical* change, more likely than not.

Again, a likely decades-long iterative process is to be expected in any country when dealing with something as complex, vast, and economically significant as healthcare. After all, we didn't put a man on the moon on our first foray into outer space. It took years and years of gradually more aggressive space excursions, some of which were unsuccessful (even with fatal consequences), before Neil Armstrong took "One small step for Man . . ." As of today, we still haven't mastered reusable, affordable, space vehicles. And, hard as it is to believe, understanding the numerous genetic and acquired illnesses and conditions that afflict our species and then sorting through the endless medications and other treatment options involves far more variables than does space exploration. Thus, it will *and should* take years filled with multiple course corrections to successfully pass through the healthcare reform storm and find ourselves on the other side: on smooth waters, with cool breezes, and blue skies. Or in real terms, to consistently experience a much healthier population and to provide healthcare of vastly greater quality and cost efficiency.

Let me also make it clear at this early point in our journey together: *this book has no specific political agenda.* In fact, we must accept that sooner-rather-than-later, one or more elected federal officials would have to risk their popularity, support, careers, and legacies by stepping up to the proverbial plate and addressing the need for meaningful healthcare reform. That by refusing to address the healthcare crisis, by simply "kicking the can down the (electoral) road," the crisis would only worsen. No, something had to be done—at least started—here and now. America had to finally at least dip our toe into the healthcare reform pool. And whether or not you agree with the initial mandated reform pathway (the ACA), you must admit that the legislation is far more than toe dipping: we're swimming now.

This book has no specific political agenda.

In looking back on previous reform attempts in America, we must seek an explanation as to why "this time is different." Why this time will reform not fade away but serve as the initiation in a challenging, continuous commitment to improve America's healthcare system? I'll offer four major reasons, *forces* (in our nautical analogy), really, which have come together at this unique time in the history of US healthcare to propel the dramatic reform movement which began soon after the 2008 US presidential election. Reform that will likely demonstrate permanency (in some form) that long outlives its designers. It is the simultaneous collision of these four major forces, in effect creating *The Perfect Healthcare Reform Storm,* that is significantly changing and will continue to significantly change how we perceive health and healthcare.

Once you understand this powerful quartet of factors behind today's irreversible reform process, we'll move on to discuss how our evolving healthcare system has changed the definition and responsibilities of THE PROVIDER, THE COIN OF THE REALM, and WHAT THE PROVIDER NEEDS to successfully function (and, hopefully, lead) in this new care environment.

So here they are, the four forces that have combined to form our *Perfect Healthcare Reform Storm . . .*

It is the simultaneous collision of these four major forces, in effect creating *The Perfect Healthcare Reform Storm,* that is changing and will continue to change how we perceive health and healthcare.

Drivers of Healthcare Reform

Now (at last!) let's dive into these four forces, the main drivers of healthcare reform.

1. Popular Acceptance That the Current Healthcare Spending Curve Is Not Sustainable

For years, it has been common knowledge among economists and politicians that our country's healthcare spending is dangerously, wildly out of control. But *public awareness and understanding (let alone concern) over the cost of healthcare* have always remained buried beneath the surface of our cumulative American subconscious, layers below other shared worries and fears about the dangers facing our nation. After all, the country's infrastructure is crumbling (an estimated 56,000 US bridges are "structurally deficient).[5] War with North Korea or Iran or Russia or somebody is always imminent. Half the country is convinced that our newly elected political leaders will "forever destroy our democracy," while the other half cries out that our outgoing legislators have "left our country in ruins." Our children have worsening math and science skills when compared with their global peers. And the stock market and unemployment… well, don't get me started!

> *Public awareness and understanding (let alone concern) over the cost of healthcare* have always remained buried beneath the surface of our cumulative American subconscious.

Thus, while economists and politicians have been acutely aware of our catastrophic healthcare spending, none of us typical Americans really paid it much attention.

Until recently.

Over the last several years, things have begun to change. *Quickly.* Financial graphs and charts depicting threatening, upward-sloping lines began to appear *outside of the pages* of *The Wall Street Journal* and the *Financial Times,* finding their way into *the lay press.* Disturbing images like Fig. 3.1 began showing up on the nightly news and in popular magazines.

Now, my 85-year-old mother may not possess a deep understanding of the meaning of this chart (that the **US National Health Expenditure** currently represents over 17% of our country's **gross domestic product [GDP]**), but Mom clearly appreciates the implications of the "Health Expenditures" line sharply heading north and that our healthcare spending has been consistently trending in this, *the wrong direction*, for decades.

Just so you (and Mom) are clear, **GDP** represents the cash value of all of the goods produced and services

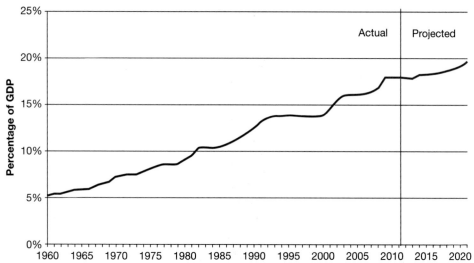

FIGURE 3.1 National health expenditures as a share of US gross domestic product (GDP).[6,7] (From Belk D. The True Cost of Healthcare. TrueCostOfHealthcare.net [online]; http://truecostofhealthcare.net/wp-content/uploads/2014/12/HealthcareGDPHistory.pdf.)

provided within the borders of a country over a specific time period (usually annually). Thus, *out of every $100 spent* on American-made products or provided services, from cell phones to groceries, from shoes to toothpaste, from carpet cleaning to pet care to dining out, *$17 are spent on healthcare-related goods and services.*

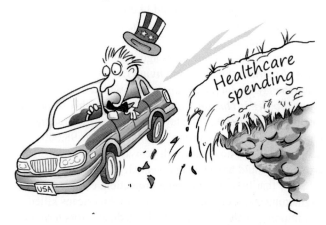

Even a first-year economics student (let alone the economic wonks who advise our political leaders) will tell you that this number, 17%, is *economically unsustainable.* That is, even if held at 17% (and that ship has sailed), such an enormous draining of cash out of our national economy leaves us with far too little to spend on education, housing, food, infrastructure, defense, or on whatever projects fit with your personal politics.

So, the first of the four forces contributing to *The Perfect Healthcare Reform Storm* is the recent heightened awareness of John and Jane Q. Public that the amount of money we are all (as a nation) spending on healthcare is rapidly approaching a very real, economically dangerous financial cliff.[8,9] And more importantly, *the general public has begun to understand that runaway healthcare spending has a direct impact on each and every one of us, as healthcare costs drive up not only individual health insurance premiums, but also lead to higher state and federal taxes, and even increase the costs of consumer goods (as employee healthcare insurance premiums continue to rise for manufacturers and retailers);* soon the public will no longer simply ignore the spiraling cost of care.

2. The Finding of a Marketable Argument

Okay, so we're spending way too much on healthcare. But hey, *you get what you pay for,* right? Obviously if we're spending so much on healthcare, *we must have the greatest healthcare in the world!* In fact, up until a few years ago, had you headed out to the nearest busy street corner and asked the first 20 people who walked by, the majority would have confidently agreed with the statement: "The United States has the best healthcare in the world." Even those who expressed less confidence would likely have acknowledged that "The United States has *one of the best* healthcare systems in the world."

At least up until a few years ago. Reality began to set in across America's kitchens and living rooms starting in 1999, when the lay media picked up and ran with a disturbing report, *To Err Is Human.* Published by the highly respected Institute of Medicine,[10] the lay media eagerly shared the report's terrifying conclusion, that "as many as 98,000 people . . . die in hospitals each year as a result of medical errors that could have been prevented."

Since that first jaw-dropping projection, even more frightening estimates of the numbers of Americans killed and injured because of preventable medical errors have been splashed across television screens and internet news sites. In 2014, wide lay press coverage exposed average Americans to much higher preventable death and injury estimates, as healthcare experts testified in front of the Senate Subcommittee on Primary Health and Aging. We watched or read in horror as these researchers now suggested that the number of Americans who died annually as a result of preventable medical errors had skyrocketed to *400,000 per year,* making preventable medical errors at the hands of well-meaning doctors, nurses, pharmacists, technicians, therapists, and other caregivers *the third leading cause of adult death* in the United States.

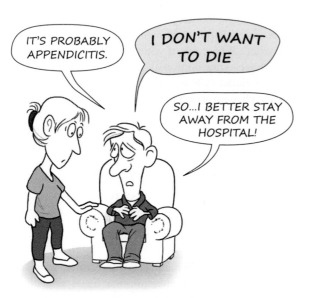

Today, debate continues to rage as to the true number of Americans killed and injured by avoidable provider mistakes. Although the actual figure of preventable patient deaths likely falls between 200,000 and 400,000,[11] *the mere introduction of such frightening numbers into the general population's consciousness has been jarring for Americans, shaking to the core our long-held confidence in our healthcare system and in the professional caregivers who provide our care.*

> Preventable medical errors are *the third leading cause of adult death* in the United States.

Nor are poor healthcare outcomes only apparent when looking at avoidable inpatient deaths. Unbelievably, *10,000 Americans suffer major preventable complications every single day,* the result of avoidable medical mistakes made by their physicians, nurses, health professionals, or other care providers.[12]

> Unbelievably, *10,000 Americans suffer preventable major complications every single day,* the result of avoidable medical mistakes.

And avoidable mistakes aren't limited to the hospital (inpatient) setting. Approximately 85% of us visit our doctor's office at least once a year. Sadly, *for greater than 5% (more than 12 million Americans), our providers either fail to correctly diagnose a condition* despite **signs, symptoms,** and/or diagnostic results (blood work, x-rays, etc.) that suggest the diagnosis, *or fail to act in a timely fashion, delaying our diagnosis.*[13]

So what? Who cares if your physician assistant misdiagnoses your bunion as a plantar wart? But what if your dietician fails to recognize that you have pre-diabetes. Or your nurse practitioner fails to diagnose your early cervical cancer? For an estimated 50% of the patients erroneously diagnosed or not diagnosed every year—that's *6 million people*—their providers' diagnostic failures have potentially serious consequences (even catastrophic, such as failing to diagnose a cancer in a timely fashion, or at all). Here's a real-world example which, no exaggeration, is similar to a story told to me by a patient every month or so:

> Don is a 59-year-old man who, during his routine annual physical examination, mentions that he occasionally sees a small amount of bright red blood on his bowel movements.
>
> "No problem," his doctor *(or nurse practitioner or physician assistant)* says reassuringly, "Lots of folks your age get hemorrhoids. Swollen blood vessels just inside the anus that can bleed if you're a bit constipated."
>
> Don nods. "Yep. I get my share of constipation," he says with a smile.
>
> "No worries," his provider says. "Try some stool softeners. You can get them over-the-counter at the drug store. Softer bowel movements usually stop the bleeding. And if not, there are simple office treatments that we can consider down the line."
>
> Indeed, many people of all ages develop hemorrhoids. One common symptom of hemorrhoids is painless, bright red blood on bowel movements or on the toilet paper, and stool softeners or additional dietary fiber can ease constipation and reduce or eliminate hemorrhoidal bleeding—which is all great.
>
> Except that Don's bleeding is not from hemorrhoids.

Nor is the true cause of Don's intermittent bleeding rare. It's *rectal cancer.* And large bowel cancer is the second leading cause of cancer deaths in American men, diagnosed in approximately 6%, of which 90% are older than 50. And rectal cancer frequently presents as intermittent, painless, limited bright red blood on bowel movements. *Just like hemorrhoids.*

That's why in Don, a 59-year-old man with intermittent bright red blood on his stools, an endoscopic evaluation of his lower large intestine (including the rectum) is required. *Demanded,* really. Even if the patient is found to have bleeding hemorrhoids, as the presence of both conditions (bleeding hemorrhoids and a bleeding rectal cancer) is not uncommon in this population.

By the time Don returns to his provider, 3 months have passed. He's back now because in addition to the bleeding (which is now more frequent despite stool softeners), Don is experiencing a new symptom. He now frequently feels like he has to move his bowels, but when he tries, "little or nothing comes out."

And he's losing weight.

Now his provider orders the diagnostic study that should have been ordered 3 months earlier, when Don first mentioned the occasional bright red blood on his stools. The colonoscopy reveals the large rectal tumor. The computed tomography (CT) scan reveals two metastases (areas where his rectal cancer has spread) in his liver . . .

What if Don's provider hadn't failed to investigate the bleeding when Don first mentioned it 3 months earlier? No doubt the rectal tumor would have been smaller. Would a CT scan have still shown the two cancer metastases in Don's liver? That is, would Don's cancer have been at a less advanced, more treatable stage? Would Don have had a better chance of not dying from his rectal cancer?

And what if Don's provider had done the right thing not 3 months ago, but *9 years ago,* when Don was 50. When his provider should absolutely have begun screening Don for colon and rectal cancer, as national guidelines recommend. Because if Don's provider followed these recommendations, then either at that first or a follow-up endoscopic screening, the benign polyp that years later would grow into this bleeding rectal cancer would have been detected and safely, swiftly, painlessly removed.

Many of the patients in my care throughout my clinical career were just like "Don." Patients whose signs and symptoms were straight out of the "How Colon and Rectal Cancer Present" section of a medical student's introductory textbook. Patients went undiagnosed or misdiagnosed by their primary care physicians, ambulatory nurses, or physician assistants despite their obvious need for large bowel diagnostic studies. Even more tragic, I frequently cared for patients who, like "Don," were never aggressively pushed (or even told) by their primary care providers to undergo the recommended large bowel cancer screening.

Why? you ask. Why would any provider fail to recommend care (including cancer screening) based on universally accepted guidelines? This is a critical question to answer, and we will answer it in Chapter 7, where we discuss the poor quality of American healthcare.

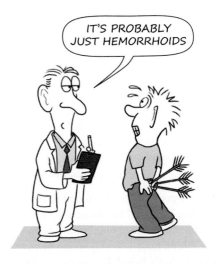

The publication of *To Err Is Human* in 1999 opened the floodgates. Soon after, the lay press was reporting on the poor quality of US healthcare on a regular basis. And the more that the lay press discussed the poor state of American healthcare, the more they also reported on the spiraling cost of US healthcare. Stories about quality and cost fed on one another (and are in reality, closely related, as quality is the numerator and cost the denominator in a useful definition of **"healthcare value"**). Over a short period of time, the general public become consciously aware that while we're spending a ridiculous amount of money on healthcare, people aren't getting high quality care. That what we are all getting in return for that 17% of our GDP is:

- Preventable medical errors are the third leading cause of adult death in the United States, killing between 200,000 and 400,000 Americans annually
- Preventable medical errors cause serious complications for 10,000 Americans each and every day
- Each year, 12 million American outpatients are erroneously diagnosed, with half of the misdiagnoses leading to potentially serious consequences

And what else have typical Americans come to appreciate? That the annual cost of diagnosing and treating all of the clinical consequences of these patients' preventable medical errors exceeds $1,000,000,000,000 (1 trillion).

Simply staggering . . .

So does the United States have the world's best healthcare? Or at least is ours *among* the world's best healthcare?

Sorry. Not even close. And more and more, Americans know it.

In recent years, evening news programs, popular websites, and other lay sources of information have increasingly reported the truth: that the United States ranks well below other nations by many measures of healthcare value. Widely cited examples include a 2000 World Health Organization report that ranks the United States healthcare system as the 37th best in the world[14] and a 2014 Commonwealth Fund survey that places the United States *last* among 11 wealthy nations[15] "in terms of 'efficiency, equity, and outcomes.'"

So at last, many Americans have begun to appreciate this startling and frightening reality: that *our current, traditional healthcare system often provides us at best only moderately good care (and at worst, very poor care).* And for those forces now aggressively pushing reform, *the significant fear that such public awareness of our poor quality healthcare generates is extremely marketable;* that is, this awareness is powerful in pulling the voting public onto the side pressing for major changes to our healthcare system.

> For those forces now aggressively pushing reform, *the significant fear that such public awareness of our poor quality healthcare generates is extremely marketable.*

3. Technology Allowing Everyone Easy, Rapid Access to Information

I sat there with my jaw literally hanging open. My teenage daughter sat silently on her bed, her entire being focused on the small screen of her smartphone. I had been standing at the open door to her room for 2 full minutes, my presence unnoticed, her eyes never even glancing away from the device (I could swear she hadn't even blinked). Finally, I interrupted.

"Who are you texting?"

She didn't even look up. "Emily," she replied mechanically.

Emily is her best friend, and also an avid texter.

"But . . ." I stammered. Perhaps it was the rare uncertainty in my voice, but my daughter finally looked up from her tiny screen and stared at my puzzled face. I gathered myself and continued. "But, *Emily is sitting on the bed next to you . . ."*

Indeed, Emily was sitting less than a foot away from my daughter, still silently focused on her own smartphone. As she texted my daughter. Sitting next to her.

"I know," my daughter replied matter-of-factly. "So?"

"So . . ." My world was spinning, growing dark and hazy. "So, *why don't you just talk to each other?"*

Now Emily finally looked up. The two teenagers exchanged glances, both slightly shaking their heads disapprovingly. Then, without replying to my clearly absurd question, their heads once again dropped down in unison, their eyes locking back onto their phone screens.

Let's face it: *personal technology has become as ubiquitous as air.* Toddlers are masters of tablets. Seniors pay their bills on their smart phones. A simple stroll down the sidewalk has become more dangerous than skydiving, what with all the people shuffling forward face-down, their entire focus on tweets and Instagram and Snapchat. (All kidding aside, search the internet for *selfie-related deaths.*)

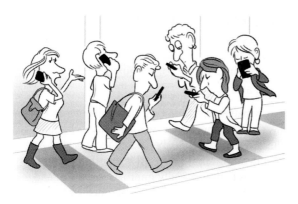

While many of us worry that there will be consequences for our children in terms of interpersonal skills and live communication competence as a result of our obsession with smart technology, there clearly are countless benefits. And healthcare has started to share in these benefits as the industry has finally begun to creep its way into the 21st century. Today, potential patients can compare hospitals and even individual physician outcomes online, all from the comfort of their own home. The idea behind such comparison sites is to provide information that allows patients to assess and compare important healthcare metrics and outcomes, from simple questions (physician office locations; medical school; years in practice; office hours) to the complex (surgical wound infection rates; procedural expertise). Powerful technology allows patients to easily communicate in real time with nurses and other providers as well as ask questions, send images, and schedule visits. Telemedicine is increasingly allowing patients the world over to have live access to provider experts oceans away.

Today, patients and their loved ones have easy, rapid access to a multitude of sites and sources offering medical information and guidance that are available in a variety of languages, educational levels, and formats. Even elderly people more often than not can quickly navigate to images of medications, allowing them to compare the pill in their hand with a large, high-definition image on their mobile phone. And those just diagnosed with virtually any condition can rapidly and easily find information, statistics, flow-charts, images, and figures about their disease, empowering them in their own care decisions. (Of course, a critical concern with all of this rapid, simple access is guiding patients to *current, credible,* and *objective* information resources, and to find information *appropriately specific* to their own disease and disease stage.)

Today, patients and their loved ones have easy, rapid access to a multitude of sites and sources offering medical information and guidance, available in a variety of languages, educational levels, and formats.

So now patients have in their hands the incredible power of easy, rapid technology. At work. At play. Anytime, anywhere. We have suddenly entered the world of *Star Trek* and in doing so, we have all been offered infinite opportunities to dramatically improve our health and healthcare. No longer is healthcare defined by "the doctor-patient relationship." Now and forever moving forward, patients and their loved ones will have information, advice, recommendations, and guidance literally at their fingertips, empowering them to play an increasingly active role in their health and healthcare decisions.

4. An Appreciation of Healthcare Economics

I remember the first time my wife and I went shopping for a home. We found a beautiful house. Plenty of space. Great layout. Big back yard for our (future) children. Close to work. It was everything we dreamed of. And it was entirely out of our reach financially.

I remember my first car. I had wanted a new Pontiac Firebird. A cool, sleek, muscle car. After all, I was a single, red-blooded, pre-med student living in sunny California. What better way to cruise my university than in a new gold Firebird? It all added up! Except when I looked at my bank statement, where none of it added up. After which I begged my parents. Based on their response, I bought a 6-year-old used Honda Accord. Which I kept for another 6 years. *Because that's what I could afford.* (In the end, the passenger door was held closed via a rope tied from the door handle to the back of the driver's seat, which didn't keep out the freezing Midwestern wind.)

We all understand the basics of American capitalism: *better quality costs more.* Want a nicer house? *It costs more.* A new Firebird instead of a used Accord? *Pay up.* A five-star four-course dinner rather than a burger and fries? *Lots more bucks.* And overall, this American economic model makes sense to us. *A "better" product or a service costs more.*

But as pointed out in discussing the first two of the four forces that have combined to form our *Perfect Healthcare Reform Storm,* the US healthcare system is not working in accordance with the American economic model. In our traditional healthcare system, Americans are getting care that is far *(far)* from the best in terms of quality, and we are paying way, way more than we should (and way, way more than can be sustained). That means that our traditional fee-for-service reimbursement model fails to align with the rest of the American economic system. *Fee-for-service has given us poorer quality that costs more.*

So how do we align our healthcare system with the rest of our economy? That is, how can we get healthcare to the point that *better care* is what costs more?

But here's the amazing thing. The dirty little secret that every caregiver knows, but which the general public is only now recognizing: *in healthcare, better quality costs less.*

Let me say that again: *IN HEALTHCARE, BETTER QUALITY COSTS LESS.*

What?! What am I saying? It's . . . it's . . . *un-American!*

Take a breath, Patriot, and think about it. Remember my earlier example in which I committed a preventable error during surgery, and then the intensive care unit (ICU) nurse made an avoidable error in medication dosing? Remember that while *the quality of care was terrible, all of the care, including the extensive, expensive care required to treat the consequences of the two preventable medical errors, was paid for.* However, had the surgery and subsequent postoperative care been appropriate (that is, without avoidable mistakes), *that "better care" would have cost much less.*

Again, *the provision of lower quality healthcare costs more.* **The provision of higher quality healthcare costs less.**

And *"better care costs less"* doesn't just apply to hospitalized patients. The potential impact of understanding and also utilizing this inverse economic reality outside of the hospital is enormous. For example, screening to prevent colorectal cancer and removing a precancerous polyp is obviously "better" for a person than developing bowel cancer. But multiple studies have also concluded that colorectal cancer screening is *cost-effective as well.*[16,17] Another example is the seasonal (annual) flu. Everyone has had it, and everyone knows how miserable it is to suffer the fevers, chills, muscle aches, coughing, and sore throat. However, due to aggressive campaigns by the Centers for Disease Control (CDC) and other public health agencies, pretty much everyone knows that they should get that little flu shot each and every year. And the shot is available everywhere: at our provider's office, at the local pharmacy, and even at your workplace. But the flu is more than just a miserable week or two slumped on the couch, it can be seriously dangerous:

- According to the CDC, hundreds of thousands of Americans are hospitalized, and tens of thousands die annually as a result of the seasonal flu (usually due to flu-related complications, such as pneumonia or heart attack).[18]

Not only can the flu vaccine prevent the misery and potential serious complications that can accompany the flu, the annual shot is cost-effective for America as a whole:

- The CDC states that the annual costs of direct care for patients with the flu and flu-related complications exceeds $10 billion.[19]

So that little needle prick provides good quality (even life-saving) benefits and is cost-effective (benefiting all of us) as well. Yet:

- The CDC findings reveal that more than 50% of Americans each year make the conscious decision *not to be vaccinated* for the flu.

These bullet points are supported by multiple studies[20,21] that leave us to clearly conclude that if all of our fellow citizens simply rolled up a sleeve and got their flu shots every year, we'd all save a heck-of-a-lot of our hard-earned money.

The provision of lower quality healthcare costs more. **The provision of higher quality healthcare costs less.**

I'll say it again: *better quality care (better outcomes for patients) costs less (for all of us).*

For decades (longer, really), doctors, nurses, and allied health professionals have all understood this economic truth. That preventable medical errors cost our patients in terms of quality of life and cost all of us dollars. But it's been kept secret. Not intentionally (unless you are a conspiracy theorist who believes that providers and hospitals *want* people to get sick in order to make money), but because the public was not yet aware of the four forces at a level to support major reform of the US healthcare system. Simply said, there was no reason for caregivers to point out that better care should cost less. In fact, it made sense for providers and hospitals *not* to point it out, as we were all aggressively practicing defensive medicine, wasting enormous amounts of money without improving care outcomes (as previously discussed).

However, this is changing. The cat is out of the bag, as the general public has slowly been let in on this powerful secret, that better quality costs less. And the subsequent recognition that our traditional fee-for-service model is not only antiquated, but *antithetical to the concept of high quality, cost efficient healthcare.* Armed with this burgeoning appreciation of how the economics of healthcare really work, the American public is understandably growing more supportive of healthcare reform.

The Four Forces Collide: Where Things Get Complicated

So there we have it, The Perfect Healthcare Reform Storm. From the north, Popular Acceptance that the Current Healthcare Spending Curve is Not Sustainable. From the south, The Finding of a Marketable Argument. From the east, Technology Allowing Everyone Easy, Rapid Access to Information. And from the west, An Appreciation of Healthcare Economics.

But how these four forces collide and interact with one another is not always simple or clean. Without better appreciating the complexities of these interactions, we will not maximize the potential for improved health and healthcare. We'll start by focusing on the relationship between our unsustainable *Healthcare Spending Curve* (greater than 17% of GDP) and the *Marketable Argument* (Americans are provided poor quality care). We'll conclude by diving deeper into the challenges of our widely available, empowering *Technology.*

Cost-of-Care Versus Quality

How do we reconcile these intuitively opposing realities: that we are spending an enormous amount for healthcare, and yet the quality of that purchased care is poor? I mean, how can we be paying through the nose for healthcare that likely can't even *treat* a bleeding nose? *How is it possible that we're paying way too much for way too mediocre care?*

The truth is that our unsustainable healthcare spending is *not the cause* of our poor health and healthcare, *it is the result* of our poor health and healthcare.

◉ PEARL

Four forces have come together at this point in time, creating *The Perfect Healthcare Reform Storm:*

1. *Popular Acceptance That the Current Healthcare Spending Curve is Not Sustainable*
2. *The Finding of a Marketable Argument* (the general public's increasing awareness that the quality of American healthcare is poor)
3. *Technology Allowing Everyone Easy, Rapid Access to Information*
4. *An Appreciation of Healthcare Economics* (a growing understanding by average Americans that in healthcare, better quality should cost less)

So if our poor health and healthcare are the *drivers* of our unsustainable spending, it makes sense to examine the factors leading to that poor quality.

The truth is that our unsustainable healthcare spending curve is *not the cause* of our poor health and healthcare, *it is the result* of our poor health and healthcare.

According to the **Centers for Disease Control and Prevention (CDC),** more than one of every three Americans meets the medical definition of "obesity.[22]" The CDC also notes that chronic obstructive pulmonary disease (COPD), a condition resulting from cigarette smoking, affects from 3% to greater than 9% of Americans, varying by state.[23] Oh yeah, and there are over 29 million type 2 diabetics in America right now (the CDC also projects that there are another 8 million with type 2 diabetes moving through their daily lives undiagnosed).[24] Remember, obesity, COPD, and type 2 diabetes, like dozens of other major health problems, are *man-made,* the result of behavioral choices. Neanderthals didn't suffer kidney failure from type 2 diabetes. Neanderthals didn't need inhalers for their chronic smokers' bronchitis. Neanderthals weren't too fat to fit into their bearskin pants.

Sorry…the truth is painful. But it's the truth nonetheless. *As a general population, Americans are terrible at avoiding behaviors that damage our health.*

Obesity, COPD, and type 2 diabetes, like dozens of other major health problems, are *man-made*, the result of behavioral choices. Neanderthals didn't suffer kidney failure from type 2 diabetes.

But what about the hundreds of diseases that *aren't the result of our behavioral choices,* that aren't "our fault?" Diseases and conditions that occur spontaneously, the consequence of genetic mutations and other factors that (at least for now) are out of our control? Turns out that *Americans also voluntarily ignore or avoid recommendations to prevent or control spontaneously acquired illnesses.* For example, CDC data reveal that one-third of American adults fail to undergo recommended colorectal cancer screening,[25] despite unavoidable, aggressive public awareness campaigns that have educated the population to the figures:

- Colorectal cancer is one of the leading cancer killers
- Roughly 1 of every 20 Americans will be diagnosed with colorectal cancer

- Screening is safe, simple, and saves lives
- Screening is covered by both private and governmental health insurance

And still, one out of three Americans simply does not undergo screening, a percentage far too great to blame on lack of awareness and/or the failure of all providers to recommend screening.

And the excuses. "The prep is awful! That liquid you have to drink tastes like sweat!" Yeah . . . surely colon surgery, chemotherapy, radiation, or death couldn't possibly be worse than drinking a jug of salty water every 5 to 7 years.

How about the annual flu shot? You don't have to drink anything, salty or otherwise. You don't have to miss a day of work. Heck, you don't even have to visit your doctor's office because flu shots are offered at virtually every drug and grocery store. In fact, many workplaces now offer on-site flu shots, so you don't even have to leave the office to avoid 2 weeks of infectious misery. Providers even joke that the only way to really avoid getting your annual flu shot is to run faster than the nurse chasing you down the street. And please don't argue that flu shots are too expensive. A shot costs most of us only a few bucks. And for many, it's free.

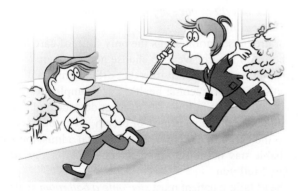

And yet as we've previously discussed, every year, more than 50% of all Americans actively choose not to be vaccinated. No biggie, right? After all, *it's only the flu.* And as we've previously discussed, every year "only the flu" *kills tens of thousands of Americans and lands hundreds of thousands in the hospital,* the result of dangerous complications of "only the flu," such as pneumonia and heart attack. This is another clear example of *our poor quality healthcare choices driving our dramatically elevated healthcare costs.*

Because of another basic truth: in general, Americans are horrible when it comes to complying with recommendations aimed at protecting our health.

Our poor quality healthcare choices drive our dramatically elevated healthcare costs.

All right. What about *once we have a disease or condition?* Faced with symptoms (pain, foot ulcers, shortness of breath, fatigue, chronic coughing, failing eyesight, etc.), do we *then* (at last) do what we can to hold our illnesses in check and keep our diseases from progressing and landing us in the emergency room, the hospital, or an even worse (and much colder) place?

No.

Let's start with medications. Fortunately, today we have an ever-growing war chest filled with wonder drugs designed to combat an enormous range and variety of ailments that plague us. And yet many of us continue to take lousy care of ourselves: *over 50% of us fail to take our prescription medications as instructed,*[26] and *more than 28% of us with chronic conditions fail to even pick up our newly prescribed medication* after leaving our provider's office.[27] In other words, even when we are suffering from our pathologies, *we often choose not to take the prescription drugs that we know can reduce or relieve our symptoms and control, slow, or even cure our illnesses.*

Nor are prescription drugs the only form of care that we choose to ignore. We also choose not to adhere to often simple and safe activities that offer significant protection from worsening health. For example, do you know what a heart failure patient must do each and every day to avoid sudden shortness of breath, an ambulance ride to the ER, a likely emergency hospital admission with a probable stay in the ICU, and even death? It's a *great burden,* I tell you.

A heart failure patient must *step onto a bathroom scale every day.*

Yep. That's the burden. Remembering to weigh themselves at the same time every morning. It takes all of 15 seconds, and other than stubbing one's toe on the scale, it's entirely without risk. You see, a subtle weight increase is a very early sign of acutely worsening heart failure and often precedes severe symptoms requiring hospitalization by several days.[28] Thus, discovering a weight increase allows the patient to seek outpatient evaluation and medication adjustment,[29] which frequently can improve the acute cardiac decompensation, allowing the patient to avoid the terrifying symptoms as well as the ER, the hospital, the ICU, and even the Grim Reaper. Talk about a win-win activity. No risk, only seconds to complete, and a tremendous health upside.

Yet heart failure remains a leading cause of hospitalization in the United States, resulting in over 1 million hospital admissions annually.[30] In addition, greater than 20% of heart failure patients are readmitted to a hospital within 30 days of a hospital discharge.[31] Hard to believe that all of these folks actually step on their bathroom scales every morning. Because (obviously) *they don't.*

How about the worldwide epidemic of type 2 diabetes, that classic man-made disease that results from too many cookies and too much time on the couch. Diabetes is a condition that attacks multiple body organs and functions. The heart, the kidneys, the arteries, the nerves, the eyes, the immune system, the brain…all are targets of this destructive disease, one of the top 10 killers.[32] Fortunately, closely monitoring blood sugar levels allows patients and their providers to control and potentially slow down the damage that the disease inflicts on the patient's body and health. But any provider knows from personal experience that many (perhaps most) diabetics don't stick to their prescribed blood sugar monitoring routine. How do we know? *They tell us.* And if they don't, we see their elevated levels of hemoglobin A1c (a circulating substance that tells us the patient's average blood sugar level over the previous several months). They routinely "forget" or skip routinely performing the safe, quick, critical finger sticks, knowing full well that *they will be the ultimate victims* of their poorly controlled disease.

Leading us to yet another truth: in general, *Americans are awful when it comes to complying with recommendations aimed at maintaining and controlling conditions that clearly threaten their health.*

So there we have it. Put it all together and we're left with one clear conclusion: *we are an unhealthy nation.* We make behavioral choices fully aware that we are injuring our bodies and our health. We voluntarily avoid activities that we are fully aware would benefit our bodies and our health. We make excuses. We play the helpless victim. We disconnect our behaviors and choices and inactions from recognized, harmful, even life-threatening consequences.

We are unhealthy.

So there we have it. Put it all together and we're left with one clear conclusion: *we are an unhealthy nation.*

Now, such a statement is, of course, a generalization. Many affluent communities experience high quality health and healthcare, whereas health and healthcare quality for less affluent individuals is poorer.[33,34] But as a *population,* as the American society in general, we all feel the impact (at least financially) of the overall low quality of health and healthcare across our nation.

Now let's bring this all back around to the theme of this section: reconciling our unsustainable healthcare spending and our nation's poor health. The answer is clear. *An unhealthy population means really, really expensive healthcare.* Thus, to reduce our already overblown-and-still-advancing healthcare spending (which we must), then the answer is to address the source of this cost explosion: improve both our health and our healthcare. And if we are ever to realize true quality health as a population (or a species), we must undertake a radical transformation. We must undergo a paradigm shift in accepting who is truly and ultimately accountable and responsible for all health and healthcare decisions, from disease prevention to continuing care to end-of-life decisions: *the patient.*

Awareness that this philosophical U-turn, placing health and healthcare "ownership" squarely on the shoulders of individual Americans lies at the root of the *Patient Engagement* movement. The concept, strategy, and tactics of successful Patient Engagement are complex, deserving of an entire chapter, which you'll find in Chapter 6. For now, suffice it to say that *unless individuals accept "health ownership," we will never realize true high-quality health, nor adequately gain control of our healthcare costs.*

> *Unless individuals accept "health ownership," we will never realize true high quality health, nor adequately gain control of our healthcare costs.*

Although patient engagement is critical to healthcare reform, engagement alone will not turn around our poor national health or the associated excessive costs of care. Patients, health professionals, nurses, doctors, *all of us must experience a paradigm shift in how we view healthcare.* That required paradigm shift includes *the uniform acceptance that today's healthcare must move away from reactive, acute care* (in which we wait for a person to become ill or grow more ill before aggressively treating that episode of illness, often in the hospital, urgent care, or ER) *to proactive, out-of-hospital preventive and maintenance care.*

Today's healthcare must move away from reactive, acute care to proactive, out-of-hospital preventive and maintenance care.

It is the combination of engaged patients who "own their health" with a societal view that health and healthcare should be proactive and primarily out-of-the-hospital that can be major drivers of higher quality and thus cost-effective care. But even this is not enough because how are engaged patients and providers to know what represents "the best care?" The answer (and another critical element of today's reform) is *evidence-based care.* To the extent possible, disease prevention, screening, and maintenance care recommendations should not be based in subjective beliefs or "professional best guesses," but on the results of solid, scientific clinical studies and trials, which through rigorous design and statistical analyses conclude (or at least strongly suggest) that *there is the clear likelihood of meaningful benefit in terms of patient quality of life and/or survival and/or cost-effectiveness if specific prevention, screening, and maintenance care guidelines are followed.* Today, evidence-based care is increasingly at the foundation of recommendations for numerous diseases and conditions: vaccinations[35] against common and/or dangerous infections; screening for breast,[36] colorectal,[37] cervical,[38] and (in a defined sub-population) lung[39] cancer; maintenance care to control or slow the progression of heart disease, diabetes, Alzheimer's disease, kidney disease. These are but a few of the thousands of illnesses and conditions for which evidence-based care clearly or likely benefits both patient and payer (the latter at the individual, national, and societal levels). (It is worth noting that many patient advocates argue for a broader *evidence-informed* care approach, which incorporates scientific evidence, provider experience, and other factors.[40])

> **PEARL**
>
> Improving the health of our population demands *Patient Engagement,* based on a dramatic paradigm shift in how we as a society view accountability and responsibility for our health and healthcare (discussed in detail in Chapter 6).

To the extent possible, disease prevention, screening, and maintenance care recommendations should not be based in subjective beliefs or "professional best guesses," but on the results of solid, scientific clinical studies and trials [evidence-based care].

So if all of these evidence-based healthcare recommendations and guidelines are available for our providers, *why is our healthcare so poor?* Yes, we've already discussed the need to engage people to own their health, but certainly providers comply with all of the available patient care evidence.

Unfortunately, this is not the case. You must understand, *just because a certain care activity is recommended doesn't mean that a healthcare provider will follow that recommendation.* Even evidence-based care guidelines are much less frequently recommended to patients by providers than they should be (even simple, inexpensive, recommendations such as daily weights for patients with heart failure). It is all too common for a cancer patient to sadly share that their providers never recommended standard screening. Even vaccinations, such as those that prevent the human papilloma virus (HPV) infections that cause virtually all cervical and most oropharyngeal (mouth and throat) cancers, are frequently never even mentioned to the parents of pediatric patients of vaccine-appropriate age during provider visits.

Over and over and over again, we find providers of all types failing to mention, to suggest, to advise, to recommend, or to strongly urge patients to engage in care activities that the evidence shows will clearly benefit their health and, consequently, the cost of healthcare.

What? Why would providers choose to ignore evidence supporting care that can improve their patients' quality of life, that might even save their patients' lives, and that will subsequently slow our runaway healthcare spending? That's . . . *that's like ignoring a red light at an intersection.*

> *Just because a certain care activity is recommended doesn't mean that a healthcare provider will follow that recommendation.*

No, it's not at all like ignoring a red light at an intersection. There are several very significant differences. The more accurate driving analogy is this: you drive up to an intersection where there are *180 different traffic lights.* Some red circles, some yellow arrows. Some flashing, some solid. Several are green. Some have silhouette figures of walking pedestrians, others solid Xs.

> Over and over and over again, we find providers of all types failing to mention, to suggest, to advise, to recommend, and to strongly urge patients to engage in activities that the evidence shows will clearly benefit their health.

In this more realistic analogy, the 180 streetlights, all of varying light patterns, symbols, and colors, represent the input the provider "driver" must consider before moving through the intersection (that is, before making a care decision). The lights include: *evidence-based information, recommendations, and guidelines; what the provider learned during training; the provider's own professional experiences; advice from colleagues; personal judgment; patient preferences; the threat of malpractice litigation; available resources; time pressure; etc.*

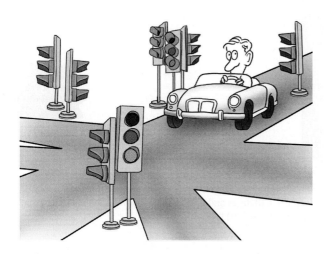

That's a whole lot for any one provider to routinely consider when making patient care decisions throughout each and every day.

Think I'm exaggerating? Listen to this stunning statistic that is only about the volume of evidence-based care information (that is, it doesn't include training, professional judgment, patient preferences, etc.)[41]:

By 2020, everything humankind knows about the body, health, and healthcare will double every 73 days.

Stop and reread that last statement. Allow the enormity, the absurdity of it to really soak in.

The pace of growth in our health and healthcare knowledge is unparalleled by any knowledge gain in all of human history (Fig. 3.2), this explosion is triggered by the revolution in our understanding of **genomics** (the human **genome**; our **DNA**).

Holy cow! Even if today's nurses, health professionals, physicians, and other care providers weren't increasingly overwhelmed with too many patients, too much documentation, too many meetings, too many phone calls, it would simply be impossible for even the most brilliant provider to master the staggering volume of medical knowledge (even the subset relevant to the provider's routine practice), let alone keep up with this explosive rate of information growth.

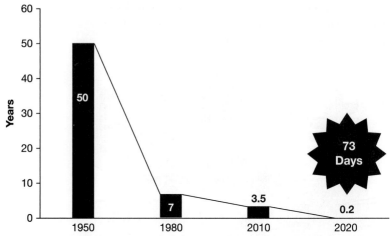

FIGURE 3.2 The trend in Doubling Time of All Medical Knowledge, 1950–2020. (From Densen P. Challenges and opportunities facing medical education. *Trans Am Clin Climatol Assoc.* 2011;122:48–58.)

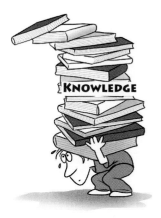

Is it surprising that today's providers seldom are willing to step away from their barely manageable clinical schedules and hectic professional lives to search for the most recently published article on patient care? Of course not. Because today, *time is the new* COIN OF THE REALM.

So *unless a health professional, nurse, or doctor is truly uncertain about the next appropriate diagnostic or therapeutic step, and only if making the wrong decision is associated with potentially serious patient risks, it is simply not worth the provider's extremely valuable time to seek additional information to confirm what the provider already suspects is "the best care."* It is much more time-effective for that provider to simply base the next care decision on their training, on what's worked before (their professional experience), on what they've heard works, or simply on what their gut tells them.

(And for the sake of simplicity, I have chosen here to avoid another very real pitfall of having all of this information available: sometimes recommendations from different, equally credible sources are in conflict. In our crazy intersection analogy, sometimes there are green lights directing opposing cars into one another.)

Today, *time is the new* COIN OF THE REALM.

So, what is the ultimate impact of too much evidence-based information (which continues to grow at a phenomenal rate) for any one provider to master?

The provision of tremendously variable patient care.

In a word, *variability* *is the single greatest obstacle to the consistent and sustainable delivery of high-quality, cost-efficient healthcare.* There is simply far, far too much information being discovered and new care guidance being generated for providers to learn, let alone utilize. The result is that *the same patient with the same medical issues will frequently undergo different diagnostic testing and/or therapeutic treatments from different providers.* Even from different providers who work within the same healthcare practice.

> In a word, *variability* *is the single greatest obstacle to the consistent and sustainable delivery of high quality, cost-efficient healthcare.*

A simple aviation analogy may suffice to clarify my ramblings:

> Deanna has wanted to fly since she was a little girl. She used to dream of flying, of soaring above the treetops. And now, at last, as a young adult, Deanna is fulfilling her dream.
>
> She once again sits in the little seat next to her flight instructor, Roy, in the cramped cockpit. She's been learning to fly, always training in the same two-seater, single-propeller plane, always under Roy's careful instruction and guidance. This is her last lesson, and once again, it is a sunny, clear Texas day, as it always has been when Deanna and Roy have flown together. She's never flown through even a light mist, let alone a rainstorm. Nor has she ever sat at the controls during a night flight.
>
> This is all fine and well, as Deanna plans to soon take her best friend on a short, daytime trip in an identical single-propeller plane. And only if the forecast calls for sunny, clear skies.

Now replace our pilot with a provider (an allied health professional, nurse, doctor, or any provider). Provider Deanna likely delivers high quality, cost-efficient care to the majority of her patients, patients who are similar to those she saw during her healthcare training under the instruction and guidance of an experienced, senior provider. These patients have diseases and needs with which Deanna is comfortable.

But the reality of healthcare, as in air travel, is this: Deanna will never know if she'll need to fly during the day or through the darkness of night; she must be able to safely fly in rain and in snow as well as on clear, sunny days; and most challenging, on some days Deanna will fly that single-propeller plane she is so comfortable with, but on others

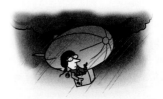

Deanna will need to fly a jet, pilot a balloon, guide a blimp, and soon, captain a spaceship.

Healthcare is so broad and so deep in its complexity that it is *simply impossible for any individual nurse, allied health professional, pharmacist, physician, or other provider to always deliver the most current, highest quality, most cost-efficient care without powerful tools* allowing for immediate access to targeted information specific to the provider and patient's needs (more on this, WHAT THE PROVIDER NEEDS, soon).

> It is *simply impossible for any individual nurse, health professional, pharmacist, physician, or other provider to always deliver the most current, highest quality, most cost-efficient care without powerful tools* allowing for immediate access to targeted information specific to the provider and patient's needs.

Here is an actual example to further clarify my meaning:

Recently, a friend e-mailed me an image of a wound on her mother's ankle, asking for my medical advice. (I've cared for a variety of foot and lower leg wounds.) My friend provided me with her mother's health history, including details about the evolution of this new, ulcerating wound. Based on this information and the photo, I suggested that it was likely a venous stasis ulcer (a skin breakdown resulting from chronic valve failure within the veins of the leg).

My friend was clearly relieved. They had already seen three physicians, two of whom had also diagnosed the wound as a venous stasis ulcer. One had recommended initial conservative nonsurgical treatment (which has been demonstrated to successfully treat many such ulcers). I agreed with this initial treatment advice. The second physician offered the same diagnosis but suggested a much more aggressive nonsurgical treatment: hyperbaric oxygen treatment, a series of lengthy "dives" in an enclosed tank which increases the amount of oxygen in the bloodstream. This expensive therapy is typically considered in certain cases where initial therapy has failed to heal the wound. The third doctor diagnosed the wound as an entirely different condition: a diabetic foot ulcer (a skin breakdown that occurs in diabetics as a result of poor arterial blood flow), despite that fact that my friend's mother has never been diagnosed with diabetes, nor is examination of the wound truly consistent with a diabetic foot ulcer. This doctor recommended beginning with an invasive diagnostic test (angiography, which is painful, costly, and carries some risk).

Remember: *this is a true story* (and, sadly, not an uncommon one).

Three doctors had all examined the same woman's ankle ulcer over a short period of time. All three had heard the exact same history. All three possessed identical information. Yet the result was *two different diagnoses,* and even the two physicians in agreement had recommended *vastly different treatments.* And the third had recommended an aggressive diagnostic study prior to any treatment.

For my friend and her mother, the questions were simple: *whose diagnosis is right, and what is the "best" treatment?*

For our healthcare system as a whole, there is a much more significant question to answer: *how do we address this variability which results in far too many poor quality outcomes and far too much financial waste?*

Because *variability is a killer, both literally and financially.*

We know this. And we know that the variability in how providers of all types deliver patient care is in large part due to their inability to sort through and utilize the mountains and mountains of evidence-based patient care information that continues to grow daily.

> *Variability is a killer, both literally and financially.*

As I shared with you already, one simply has to look at the numbers to appreciate the devastating impact that the variability in care provided by America's doctors, nurses, and allied health professionals has on us all:

- Preventable medical errors are the *third leading cause of adult death* in the United States, estimated as killing between 200,000 and 400,000 Americans annually.
- Preventable medical errors cause serious complications for *10,000 Americans each and every day.*
- Each year, *12 million American outpatients are erroneously diagnosed,* with half of these mistakes potentially leading to serious health consequences for the patient.

Even if we choose to ignore the monumental personal pain, suffering, and reduction in quality of life, simply choosing to focus on the actual *monetary costs* of our variable healthcare, here's the disastrous reality:

- *The annual direct and indirect financial cost of preventable medical errors in the United States is approximately $1,000,000,000,000 (yes, that's a whopping 1 trillion dollars).*[42]

And that's just the cost of preventable medical errors. Add to this *the failure of providers to recommend* the most appropriate preventive care activities (screenings, vaccinations, routine exams, etc., etc.) and maintenance care behaviors (daily weight checks, routine blood glucose monitoring, etc.), and it's actually surprising that we spend *only 17% of our gross domestic product* on healthcare.

No doubt the continuing explosion in healthcare knowledge offers us an enormous opportunity to improve both our health and our healthcare delivery, not just in the United States, but across the world, and in doing so, to slow runaway healthcare spending. But it is a classic double-edged sword, because there is too much to learn for any one provider to remain current on care recommendations and because the learning process must be continuous. Thus, we're left with dramatic variability in healthcare delivery, even care for those with common diseases and conditions. And while the delivery of healthcare is variable, the result of this variability is uniform: *healthcare which is both suboptimal in quality and is a main driver of our out-of-control healthcare spending.*

> ### ● PEARL
>
> The poor quality of American healthcare is largely *the result of significant variability* in how providers practice care delivery, which itself is heavily due to *the suffocating quantity of expanding, evidence-based information.* Addressing this variability challenge is critical to successful reform (and is discussed in upcoming chapters, especially Chapter 7).

The Challenges of Technology

The third force, *Technology Allowing Everyone Easy, Rapid Access to Information,* seems to be wonderful and flawless. Current, credible, evidence-based information at every patient's fingertips. *Rapidly accessible. Easy to understand.* Text, graphs, charts, images. *Everything patients need* right on their tablets or smartphones.

It's like having all of the nutritional facts right there in plain black and white labels stuck onto the boxes and jars and cans that line our grocery store shelves!

Except that it's *not* as simple as our food labels, because presenting complex healthcare outcomes data to a general population possessing widely varying levels of education and insight poses enormous challenges not faced by food manufacturers when presenting "grams of fat per serving." Here's an actual, recent, real-world example:

Academic Hospital is widely regarded as among the top ten cardiac surgery centers in the world and as the #3 cardiac care facility in America. Home to top-tier heart surgeons, cardiologists, and some of the most innovative and cutting-edge researchers, Academic Hospital is understandably proud of its reputation.

Only a few miles down the road sits Community Hospital. Providing solid quality heart care, Community Hospital is well regarded locally but certainly has no regional (let alone national or global) reputation as a cardiac surgery Center of Excellence.

Thus, when the first on-line, "objective" ranking of regional cardiac surgery centers was released, it was no small wonder that the folks at Academic Hospital went berserk.

According to the regional cardiac surgery center rankings on the government-provided website, Community Hospital was the second best cardiac surgery center in the region. And Academic Hospital?

Number 5.

Number 5! How could this be? How could an impartial, credible website offering objective cardiac surgery patient outcomes get it so wrong? How could patients be so dramatically misled?

As they say, "the devil is in the details." One of the great challenges in providing "objective" outcomes data to the general population involves *data stratification and weighting.* An understanding of how the website staff analyzed the patient outcomes data provides the explanation for what actually led to these inverted hospital rankings (and a warning on the dangers of data presentation).

It is without debate that heart surgery patients at Community Hospital suffered *fewer deaths and serious complications* than did cardiac surgery patients at Academic Hospital. But the key question is, *why*? Because, as a general community medical center, Community Hospital and its physicians and staff focus on *caring for "routine" heart disease patients and performing much less complicated and risky cardiac surgical procedures.* Whenever a high risk patient wanders into the Community Hospital ER (e.g., someone who has previously undergone open heart surgery, or someone whose heart valve suddenly fails), or if it is determined that a Community Hospital inpatient requires an extremely complicated heart operation, *Community Hospital (appropriately) transfers that patient to Academic Hospital.* Academic Hospital offers the highest level of heart care, accepting even the most complex patients, and markets itself as such. It is also a teaching hospital, filled with students, interns, and residents. Thus, the sickest patients and those faced with the most challenging cardiac surgical procedures are the exact patients that Academic Hospital seeks to care for.

Community Hospital is designed to care for and operate on the area's healthier, less complex heart surgery patients. Academic Hospital sits on the far end of the risk-complexity heart surgery spectrum. Such a scenario is not only common, but often beneficial to a large community, as it provides the most cost-effective yet appropriate care to all cardiac surgery patients.

So in terms of pure patient outcomes, not surprisingly, more of Academic Hospital's (high risk, complex) cardiac surgery patients die or suffer complication than do heart surgery patients cared for in Community Hospital. *Because Academic Hospital's patients are much more ill, much poorer surgical candidates, and/or need far more complicated operative procedures* than the healthier, less complicated patients cared for at Community Hospital.

By ignoring these significant *differences between the two patient populations,* the public was unaware that the website was actually comparing "apples to oranges." Many in the regional population likely assumed that the website had compared "apples to apples," patients of similar illness severity and surgical complexity. So you can imagine the potential consequences of such unintentional misguidance, for the patients, for the two hospitals, and for the payers.

How had this happened? The governmental public healthcare comparison website team had good intentions, but they faced the challenge of simplifying highly complex patient data for use by the general public. But the team believed that analyzing and presenting the complicated data to the general population in the manner presented to healthcare professionals (weighting the data, adjusting the data for severity of illness, complexity and risk of operative procedure) would lead to comparisons far too complicated for much of the lay public to understand and utilize in making care decisions. So, without even a note to explain that Academic Hospital alone possessed the skills and experience to care for the sickest, most complex heart patients (whereas Community Hospital did not), the website creators simply compared patient outcomes *as if both hospitals operated on identical populations of heart surgery patients.*

This is but one example of the significant and impactful real-world challenges that face us as we embrace *Technology Allowing Everyone Easy, Rapid Access to Information.* It's not the technology itself that's problematic, it's *what information to provide and how to provide it* that turns out to be far harder than at first imagined. It will take time for us to figure out better, more accurate ways of sharing healthcare outcomes information with our population of diverse education and language capabilities. In the meantime, even if we choose to temporarily ignore *care comparison* websites and tools, the number of resources offering accurate, clear, powerful, healthcare information to consumers continues to increase. In other words, there is plenty of credible guidance available today through our amazing, affordable technology to empower patients in moving towards better health, higher quality healthcare, and reduced care costs.

> It's not the technology itself that's problematic, it's *what information to provide and how to provide it* that turns out to be far harder than at first imagined.

Conclusions

The collision of these four driving forces to form *The Perfect Healthcare Reform Storm* is what makes this recent healthcare reform movement so unique and different from past reform attempts. This time, healthcare reform will not simply fade away. This time, we will not *(cannot)* ultimately return to the traditional fee-for-service reimbursement model. This time, physicians *cannot* "go it alone," relying only on their own training, experience, and judgment in guiding patient care. This time, nurses, therapists, pharmacists, technicians, dieticians, and all other healthcare professionals will *(must)* step up to play leading roles in the delivery of high value healthcare. This time, patients should not *(must not)* blindly accept without question whatever the provider recommends. This time, Americans *will not* continue to blindly dole out even greater portions of our paychecks to pay for variable healthcare.

We now move on to the next chapter, where we will more specifically revisit those three significant components of any healthcare system, exploring the many ways in which healthcare reform is dramatically changing THE PROVIDER, THE COIN OF THE REALM, and WHAT THE PROVIDER NEEDS.

References

1. The debate we're yet to have about private health insurance. The conversation (online) 2015; http://theconversation.com/the-debate-were-yet-to-have-about-private-health-insurance-39249.
2. Bennet CC. Are we there yet? A journey of health reform in Australia. *Med J Aust.* 2013;4:251–255.
3. Simonet D. The new public management theory in the British health care system: a critical review. *Adm Soc.* 2015;47:802–826.
4. Ham C. *Reforming the NHS from within.* The King's Fund (online); 2014. https://www.kingsfund.org.uk/sites/files/kf/field/field_publication_file/reforming-the-nhs-from-within-kingsfund-jun14.pdf.
5. Simpson I. *Almost 56,000 U.S. Bridges Structurally Deficient: report.* Reuters (online); 2017. https://www.yahoo.com/news/almost-56-000-u-bridges-structurally-deficient-report-180021347.html.
6. Catlin AC, Cowan CA. *History of Health Spending in the United States, 1960–2013.* Centers for Medicare and Medicaid Services (online); 2015. https://www.cms.gov/Research-Statistics-Data-and-Systems/Statistics-Trends-and-Reports/NationalHealthExpendData/Downloads/HistoricalNHEPaper.pdf.
7. U.S. National Health Expenditures as a Share of GDP, 1960–2021. Centers for Medicare and Medicaid. (online); http://truecostofhealthcare.net/wp-content/uploads/2014/12/HealthcareGDPHistory.pdf.
8. Auerbach David I, Kellermann Arthur L. *How Does Growth in Health Care Costs Affect the American family?* RAND Corporation (online); 2011. http://www.rand.org/pubs/research_briefs/RB9605.html.
9. Kellermann A, Auerbach D. *Health Care Cost Growth is Hurting Middle-Class Families.* Health Affairs Blog (online); 2013. http://healthaffairs.org/blog/2013/01/03/health-care-cost-growth-is-hurting-middle-class-families/.
10. *To Err is Human.* Institute of Medicine, National Academy of Science; 1999.
11. James JT. A new evidence-based estimate of patient harms associated with hospital care. *J Patient Saf.* 2013;122–128.
12. Expert Testimony Provided to the United States 2014 Senate Subcommittee on Primary Health & Aging.

13. Sing H, Meyer AN, Thomas EJ. The frequency of diagnostic errors in outpatient care: estimations from three large observational studies involving US adult populations. *BMJ Qual Saf*. 2014;23:727–731.

14. The World Health Report 2000—Health systems: improving performance. World Health Organization (online) 2000; http://www.who.int/whr/2000/en/.

15. US health system ranks last among eleven countries on measures of access, equity, quality, efficiency, and healthy lives. *The Commonwealth Fund* (online) 2014; http://www.commonwealthfund.org/publications/press-releases/2014/jun/us-health-system-ranks-last.

16. Lansdorp-Vogelaar I, Knudsen AB, Brenner H. Cost-effectiveness of colorectal cancer screening. *Epidemiol Rev*. 2011;33:88–100.

17. Patel SS, Kilgore ML. Cost effectiveness of colorectal cancer screening strategies. *Cancer Control*. 2015;22:248–258.

18. *Centers for Disease Control and Prevention* (online) 2016; https://www.cdc.gov/flu/protect/keyfacts.htm.

19. Molinari NA, Ortega-Sanchez IR, Messonnier ML, et al. The annual impact of seasonal influenza in the US: measuring disease burden and costs. *Vaccine*. 2007;25:5086–5096.

20. Nichol KL, Margolis KL, Wasi C, et al. The efficacy and cost effectiveness of vaccination against influenza among elderly persons living in the community. *N Engl J Med*. 1994;331:778–784.

21. Muennig PA, Khan K. Cost-effectiveness of vaccination versus treatment of influenza in healthy adolescents and adults. *Clin Infect Dis*. 2001;33:1879–1885.

22. *Centers for Disease Control and Prevention* (online) 2016; https://www.cdc.gov/obesity/data/adult.html.

23. *Centers for Disease Control and Prevention* (online) 2016; https://www.cdc.gov/copd/data.html.

24. *Centers for Disease Control and Prevention* (online) 2014; https://www.cdc.gov/diabetes/data/statistics/2014statisticsreport.html.

25. *Centers for Disease Control and Prevention* (online) 2013; https://www.cdc.gov/media/releases/2013/p1105-colorectal-cancer-screening.html.

26. Brown MT, Bussell JK. Medication adherence: WHO cares. *Mayo Clin Proc*. 2011;86:301–314.

27. Fischer MA, Stedman MR, et al. Primary medication non-adherence: analysis of 195,930 electronic prescriptions. *J Gen Intern Med*. 2010;25:284–290.

28. Chaudhry SI, Wang Y, Concato J, et al. Patterns of weight change preceding hospitalization for heart failure. *Circulation*. 2007;116:1549–1554.

29. Sherer AP, Freeman L, Owens D, et al. Weighing in on the facts: best practices in daily weight monitoring for heart failure patients. *Heart Lung*. 2012;41:432–433.

30. *Centers for Disease Control and Prevention* (online) 2015; https://www.cdc.gov/nchs/data/databriefs/db108.htm.

31. McLaren DP, Jones R, Plotnik R, et al. Prior hospital admission predicts thirty-day hospital readmission for heart failure patients. *Cardiol J*. 2016;23:155–162.

32. American Diabetes Association (online); http://www.diabetes.org/diabetes-basics/statistics/.

33. Cooper RA. Regional variation and the affluence-poverty nexus. *JAMA*. 2009;302:1113–1114.

34. Cooper RA. Geographic variation in health care and the affluence-poverty nexus. *Adv Surg*. 2011;45:63–82.

35. Szucs T. Cost-benefits of vaccination programmes. *Vaccine*. 2000;18:S49–S51.

36. Screening for Breast Cancer. U.S. Preventive Services Task Force 2009 (online); http://www.uspreventiveservicestaskforce.org/uspstf/uspsbrca.htm.

37. Screening for Colorectal Cancer. U.S. Preventive Services Task Force 2008 (online); http://www.uspreventiveservicestaskforce.org/uspstf/uspscolo.htm.

38. Screening for Cervical Cancer. U.S. Preventive Services Task Force 2012 (online). http://www.uspreventiveservicestaskforce.org/uspstf/uspscerv.htm.

39. Screening for Lung Cancer. U.S. Preventive Services Task Force 2013 (online). http://www.uspreventiveservicestaskforce.org/uspstf/uspslung.htm.

40. Woodbury G, Kuhnke JL. *Evidence-based practice versus evidence-informed practice: what's the difference?* ResearchGate (online); 2014. https://www.researchgate.net/publication/260793333_Evidence-based_Practice_vs_Evidence-informed_Practice_What%27s_the_Difference.

41. Densen P. Changes and opportunities facing medical education. *Trans Am Clin Climatol Assoc*. 2011;122:48–58.

42. Classen DC, Resar R, Griffin F, et al. Global trigger tool shows that adverse events in hospitals may be ten times greater than previously measured. *Health Aff*. 2011;30:581–589.

CHAPTER 4

Tossing the Traditional Healthcare Model Onto Its Head

In the last chapter, we explored the forces that have combined to drive the reform that is currently disrupting our healthcare system. In this chapter, we will dig into that reform to understand the guiding principles and outcome metrics that lie at its heart. Most importantly to you, dear reader, is that we'll now begin to view the enormous impact of reform on your roles, responsibilities, and needs. That is, we'll see how relative to the traditional healthcare system, healthcare reform has dramatically altered the three major healthcare components:

1. The Definition and Responsibilities of THE PROVIDER
2. THE COIN OF THE REALM
3. WHAT THE PROVIDER NEEDS

But before we dive deeper, understand that if we are to achieve *meaningful* healthcare reform, *we must accept and implement several major, difficult changes* in how we view our health and our healthcare. Not only allied health professionals, nurses, physicians, and others directly involved in the delivery of healthcare, but *everyone* must accept the new paradigm. *Our entire society as a whole.*

The Aim of Healthcare Reform (In a Word)

To appreciate how the three major components of healthcare are being significantly altered by attempted reform, we must first clarify the goals of reform based on all we've shared in the previous chapters. Many specifics about our reform goals are extensively covered in subsequent chapters, but for our purposes here, I'll simplify: in a nutshell, *healthcare reform is aimed at consistently and sustainably improving the value of our health and our healthcare.*

Value

It's one of those words that everyone thinks means the same thing to all of us yet actually has a different meaning for each of us. A general definition is that "value is defined as outcomes relative to costs.[1]" We can all work towards our shared healthcare improvement goals by adopting an even simpler, more specific definition in the form of an equation:

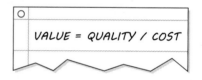

$$VALUE = QUALITY / COST$$

Want to increase the value of healthcare? *Improve the quality of care* (better patient outcomes, increased prevention, improved medication compliance, etc.).

Want to increase the value of healthcare? *Reduce unnecessary spending* (no computed tomography scan for that 8-year-old boy with obvious appendicitis, and *legislate tort reform* to dramatically reduce the practice of defensive medicine, etc.).

Really want to increase the value of healthcare? *Do both!* Drive quality improvement *and* cost reduction.

In a nutshell, healthcare reform is aimed at consistently and sustainably improving health and the value of healthcare.

But *there is great danger here.* The immediate knee-jerk reaction of many government and healthcare leaders is the assumption that the value equation runs just as easily in both directions. But while "$4 = 8 \div 2$" and "$2 \times 4 = 8$" are both equally true mathematical equations, this is the real world of healthcare. So *while it is true that better quality care costs less, it is a common and fatal mistake to also assume that the reverse is similarly true.* That is, *erroneously assuming that reducing healthcare spending will equate to improved quality.* In fact, *focusing too heavily on reducing the costs of care will risk worsening the quality of delivered care* rather than improving it, as caregivers push to cut costs by avoiding or delaying even appropriate diagnostic and/or therapeutic care activities.

I had just completed my surgical fellowship and, at 34, was finally out of training. A real surgeon. Practicing for the first time without a net. It was the mid-1990s, and yet another model of healthcare, "capitation," was spreading across the country like a virus.[2] Capitation's new structure was the Health Maintenance Organization (HMO), which were popping up everywhere, like mushrooms on rotting wood. Physicians and hospitals were in over their heads, negotiating complex care delivery contracts with far more savvy attorneys representing the interests of their clients, health insurers.

Only too late did we realize that we had signed deals with the devil. That, in fact, in our new capitation healthcare model, the best route to provider reimbursement was to *not see* patients. To *not refer* patients. To *not provide care,* because this iteration of healthcare reform was completely one-way and erroneously based on the misunderstanding of the healthcare value equation. The capitation approach to reform seemed to be all about (*only really about*) cost reduction.

And, not surprisingly, this sole focus on spending not only failed to improve the quality of care, it led to *poorer* care.

I got my first introduction to the negative quality impact of targeted cost reductions soon after entering the medical workforce. In my clinic building, a competent **primary care physician (PCP)** evaluated a 20-something-year-old who broke his ankle playing soccer with his college buddies. His insurance required that he first see his assigned PCP rather than go directly to an orthopedic surgeon, as in the capitation healthcare model of the 1990s, PCPs were designated as "gatekeepers," as their approval was required for any care referral (except for those patients willing to pay for less restrictive oversight via a more costly insurance offering). Thus the young man with the broken ankle soon found himself sitting in the office of a PCP whom he had never met but whom he had every reason to assume would offer him the very best available care.

Just like all of us who naively entered into those initial capitated contracts, the PCP in my clinic building had been learning about capitation-based healthcare the hard way: by losing money delivering care, and one of the quickest ways to lose income was for a PCP to refer a patient to a specialist.

And so it was with this PCP. Already making a limited income (relative to other physicians), still paying off medical school loans, and living and practicing in costly Southern California, he had already felt the financial sting when referring patients to specialists. *Not this time,* he decided. After all, he had trained a little in the application of splints and casts. Mind you, it was always under the guidance of a physician experienced in the care of fractures. And never for a broken ankle. But how hard could it be?

Turns out it can be very hard. Even setting and casting a complicated fracture of a long bone can be challenging if you don't really know what you're doing. And the ankle? Well, it's no long bone. The ankle is an extremely complex, multi-bone, weight-bearing joint. Trust me: if you suffer a broken ankle that's anything more than "simple fracture," see an orthopedic surgeon.

But another referral to a specialist (particularly a surgeon) would have been yet another major blow to this PCP's earnings. And again, it was only an ankle fracture.

You can imagine what happened, and you'd be right. The PCP did his best to set and cast the young man's broken ankle, which was complex in nature. Thus, not surprisingly, the PCP did not do the job correctly (or even remotely correctly). Unable to walk (let alone run, let alone play soccer) following the removal of the cast some 8 weeks later, the poor, young college student had to then undergo a series of operations (performed by an orthopedic surgeon) to correct what should have been successfully treated nonsurgically at initial presentation. And, as I recall, the damage was never fully reversed, leaving the young man with a permanent functional disability.

And the PCP with an enormous malpractice litigation settlement.

We must not allow ourselves to primarily (let alone solely) focus on driving down the cost of healthcare. Not the government, not private insurers, not politicians, not anyone. Meaningful cost reductions will occur *if we maintain the majority of our focus on improving the quality of healthcare,* on doing what's right and what's necessary for our patients, but nothing more, nothing unnecessary or of little likely benefit to our patients (difficult as that may be in the absence of tort reform). Remember our mantra: *better healthcare costs less.*

> *While it is true that better quality care costs less, it is a common and fatal mistake to also assume that the reverse is similarly true.*

Capitation-based care has faded away (although components still remain in some care models). We went back to our traditional fee-for-service approach. And now, decades later, this traditional model is once again being phased out across the country, this time in one fell swoop. But unlike capitation, the design of our new healthcare delivery model is much more consistent with the rest of the American economy: *value-based care.* As the name implies, *both the quality and the cost efficiency of care serve as the foundation of our new healthcare model, and both quality and cost efficiency play roles in determining provider reimbursement.*

Where our traditional fee-for-service model has failed (through the disconnection of quality and payment), a strong, direct link now defines our value-based healthcare model. Not surprisingly, that link is called *value-based reimbursement.* The idea of value-based reimbursement is simple: provide high-quality, cost-efficient care and you can "share in the savings;" that is, providers can earn additional money for high value care delivery. But provide low-quality, cost-inefficient care and providers will suffer *financial penalization;* that is, you (or your employer organization) will lose money.

> Meaningful cost reductions will occur if we maintain the majority of our focus on improving the quality of healthcare, on doing what's right, and what's necessary but nothing more, nothing unnecessary or of little likely benefit to our patients.

So value-based reimbursement (and through it, value-based care) relies on the old carrot-and-stick model. Unfortunately, reform legislation offers only the tiniest of carrots ("shared savings" are only a dream for the vast majority of providers) while wielding a massive stick (in the form of financial penalties).[3,4] In its first few annual cycles, the Affordable Care Act (ACA) empowered the federal government to hand out thousands upon thousands of penalties (often in the millions of dollars) to hospitals and provider organizations which failed to achieve government-defined quality standards for a number of diseases, conditions, and processes. Here are some real-world headlines:

"More Than 2200 Hospitals Face Penalties Under ObamaCare Rules[5]"

"A provision of ObamaCare is set to punish roughly two-thirds of US hospitals evaluated by Medicare starting this fall over high readmission rates…"

"Nearly 1500 Hospitals Penalized Under Medicare Program Rating Quality[6]"

"More hospitals are receiving penalties than bonuses in the second year of Medicare's quality incentive program, and the average penalty is steeper than it was last year, government records show."

"Most Hospitals Face 30-Day Readmissions Penalty in Fiscal 2016[7]"

"Only 799 out of more than 3400 hospitals subject to the Hospital Readmissions Reduction Program performed well enough on the CMS' [Centers for Medicare and Medicaid] 30-day readmission program to face no penalty…"

These are but three reports (one from 2012, one from 2013, and the last from 2016), and they are reporting on only a few of the numerous quality-based government penalty programs included in our legislated healthcare reform.

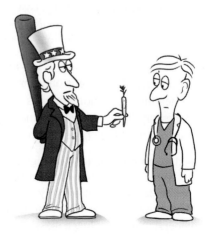

Why? Because once again, our current attempt at reform is primarily driven by a misconception: the circular logic that to improve the quality of care in those hospitals and healthcare systems which are providing poorer quality care, simply cut their revenue (through financial penalties). I struggle to think of a service for which reducing payment has dramatically improved the quality dramatically of that service. If we paid less for our air travel, do you think that the airlines would respond by improving the quality of the in-flight service? If we pay teachers lower salaries, will the quality of our children's education suddenly rise? By "following the shiny object" (cost reduction), we are yet again failing to take the best approach to healthcare value improvement. The (many) hospitals and health systems that were penalized under the new reform legislation had not been actively attempting to provide poorer quality care to their patients prior to passage of the law. Nor did they simply choose to ignore the stiff penalties codified in the reform law. So while it's true that much money in healthcare is wasted on activities that don't benefit patients (such as the practice of defensive medicine to avert medical malpractice litigation), *provider organizations that are penalized are often the very hospitals and care facilities that will be most hurt (in terms of quality of care delivery) by additional financial sanctions.* So many of today's healthcare facilities were barely surviving financially before legislated reform[8] that additional losses of revenue[9] will only further reduce the quantity and quality of care services offered.

> Where our traditional fee-for-service model has failed (through the disconnection of quality and payment), a strong, direct link now defines our value-based care model.

In reality, one reason it is so hard to improve the quality of healthcare delivery is that *it frequently takes cash investments (often significant cash investments) to build and implement processes and hire the appropriate staff necessary to increase the quality of delivered care.*

Last weekend, I brought my mother to the emergency room. She had called that day, complaining that she was "having a hard time finding some words." In fact, this difficulty was apparent during the first minutes of our phone conversation, as she would occasionally "get stuck," not losing her stream of thought, but simply unable to pull the correct word from within her brain. And, she went on to say, she had awoken hours earlier to find her left elbow and wrist "frozen in the bent position" and her left hand clenched into a fist. She was quite frightened, as she was unable to open her hand or straighten out her arm without using her functional right hand.

She assured me that she was better now (other than the word loss thing).

I told her to get dressed, and that I was on my way.

My mom had suffered at least one transient ischemic attack (TIA). TIAs are caused by decreased blood flow (thus the word "ischemic") to an area of the brain. Reversible (thus the word "transient"), they are big-time warnings that a nonreversible, major stroke may strike at any time, leaving the patient unable to speak, partially paralyzed, or worse.

TIAs are emergencies, and there is agreement on the plan of care: an emergency CT or magnetic resonance (MR) of the brain (to find evidence of a blood clot, which is treated emergently by powerful blood clot-busting agents); and if the CT shows a normal brain, then for patients such as my mom (who had paralysis of her arm for greater than 10 minutes and more than one TIA over a short period of time), an emergency ultrasound or other, more invasive study to evaluate the two large carotid arteries in the neck for evidence of obstruction of blood flow to the brain (requiring emergency surgery).

To their credit, our local ER team understood the urgency of my mother's situation (the potential for a major stroke at any time) and rapidly admitted her to the emergency room. Then they did a solid job getting her to the CT scanner within half an hour. Her brain appeared "normal for an 83-year-old woman," so the plan (recommended by her ER doctor, and with which I agreed) was to get her immediately to ultrasound in case she required an emergency operation to open the blood flow in her carotid artery.

And she did get her carotid artery ultrasound.

Ten hours later.

Because Mom had to get into the emergency radiology queue behind a dozen or so other patients waiting for their emergency ultrasounds, CT scans, magnetic resonance imaging (MRIs), and other imaging studies.

After an exasperating 10 hours (and a frightening 10 hours, as both my mother and I understood the risk she was at), I finally had an intense discussion with her hospitalist (the physician caring for her in the hospital). He had yet to see her, explaining that "the hospital has repeatedly refused to pay for additional hospitalists to care for patients during the nights," so he was responsible for more patients than he could handle. He went on to sympathize with our plight, telling us that he "had stacks of patients in real danger and in need of x-rays, but again, the hospital had refused to pay for additional radiology technicians on nights and weekends."

No doubt the hospital would plead financial stress when faced with such poor (dangerous) quality care due to limited staffing (likely not a successful argument if faced with a lawsuit). Still, this is an all-too-common, real-world example of a hospital already struggling to stay afloat financially when along comes healthcare reform to take away even more of their reimbursement dollars. One could credibly argue that to improve the quality of care, *we may actually need to initially invest more money to hire the necessary additional staff* (as well as realize tort reform to reduce unnecessary defensive medicine-associated costs of care).

In addition to the financial constraints on improving healthcare, the timeline demanded by the federal reform legislation is, in politically correct verbiage, *challenging.* Because the legislated reform timeline appears to ignore the fact that we're talking about greater than 17% of the United States' gross domestic product, impacting not only our nation's economy, but also personally affecting enormous numbers of people (patients, employees, etc.). It's like demanding that we double the number of US Naval vessels and triple the number of combat-ready Marines... by next Thursday.

How could our politicians be so foolish?

They aren't. Our politicians just live in a different world than we do. They live in a world where *calendars are aligned with elections.* The administration that drove through the ACA, that took the first plunge into true healthcare reform (whether or not you agree with that reform), created a timeline *allowing them to claim when seeking reelection* that they were action-oriented and that they had delivered a plan that promised rapid healthcare value improvement. But this politically driven healthcare policy timeline had little chance of realistically succeeding in the real world, where healthcare is vast, complex, disjointed, slow-moving.

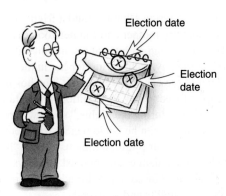

Healthcare Reform Timeline

(Here again I need to restate that I have no specific anti-reform, anti-ACA, or anti-Obama agenda. It's simply that political agendas rarely align with real-world operational agendas.)

Suffice it to say for the purposes of this book that our most recent foray into legislated healthcare reform has not been a raging success. But as I've already argued, such a complex, major economic and societal course correction will likely take years and require multiple iterations before we actually approach something resembling "success." So let's just understand the key point of the new healthcare model (and likely of any future iteration of that model): *it's all about value, for the patient (quality) and for those paying into the system (cost).*

> *It's all about value, for the patient (quality) and for those paying into the system (cost).*

The Impact of Healthcare Reform on the Definition and Responsibilities of THE PROVIDER

Reimbursement will be based on "value." Yet what is accepted as "value" and as "best practice" in healthcare will continually change, as our library of current, credible, evidence-based information continues to expand at a remarkable rate (remember, our health and healthcare knowledge will soon be doubling *every 73 days*). So to be paid (or, more realistically under the current reform legislation, to avoid major financial penalties), *providers will somehow have to keep up with the changing care activities that define "value."*

How can any one practicing doctor, or even practicing doctors as a professional population, keep current with this massive amount of continuously doubling information?

There are two parts to this answer. The first part of the answer is that *it is no longer feasible for us to view "The Doctor" alone as* THE PROVIDER.

> To be paid (or, more realistically under the current reform legislation, to avoid major financial penalties), *providers will somehow have to keep up with the changing care activities that define "value."*

That said, the overwhelming volume of healthcare information is not the only reason that our society must begin to recognize the true potential importance of nurses, allied health professionals, and other non-physicians as "providers." Much of the new information that must guide our value-based care *does not specifically relate to care provided by physicians*. One of the major impacts of reform is that *healthcare is being driven out of the hospital*,[10,11] to the medical office, even to commercial care delivery sites (think CVS and Walgreens[12]) and to the patient home.[13–15] This goal can only be achieved by *changing from reactive care* (in which we wait until someone gets really ill) *to proactive, preventive, and maintenance healthcare*. To begin this journey, nurses, allied health professionals, and many other non-physicians must take on significantly greater responsibilities if our patients are to benefit from truly value-based care (more on this soon). It is, therefore, an error to think about our growing pool of healthcare knowledge only in terms of how it can guide *physicians*. Advances in our knowledge of physical therapy, dietary practice, respiratory therapy, nursing, sonography, wound care, etc. demand that our concept of THE PROVIDER expand to include the variety of allied health professionals and nurses, as *each must keep up-to-date on "best practices" in their own area of specialization* to ensure that our patients consistently receive high value, cost-efficient care (which also ensures that their providers are reimbursed for that care).

Finally, *specialization itself demands that our provider list expand*. As we gain more valuable knowledge, much of what we are learning is highly complex and detailed, requiring trained, committed, experienced providers if we are to successfully translate newly discovered information into impactful patient care. An obvious example is the exploding field of genomics. Gene sequencing technology is advancing at an unimaginable rate.[16] It seems that every day, researchers deliver new insights into how our genes influence disease risk and treatment response and behavior. But incorporating newly discovered genetic knowledge into actual patient care requires special training, knowledge, and skills not possessed by many traditional providers (including physicians). Already, Genetic Counselors[17,18] are shouldering some of these responsibilities, helping to bring clinically impactful genomics into the patient care arena. These Genetic Counselors, along with Certified Diabetic Educators, Oncology Nutritionists, and other non-physician care specialists must also now be viewed as *full-fledged members of the provider team.*

It is no longer feasible for us to view "The Doctor" alone as THE PROVIDER.

There are also significant operational reasons for expanding the provider team, the result of our changing approach to care delivery, as we shift to out-of-hospital, consumer-focused preventive and maintenance care. For example, in the Patient-Centered Medical Home (PCMH) model,[19] the traditional doctor's office days and hours of service are greatly expanded.[20] PCMHs routinely open earlier and remain open later into the evenings. PCMHs also frequently offer appointments 6 days a week. A PCMH provider is available to speak or email patients 24/7/365. PCMHs often also dramatically increase the number of primary care patients per physician (the "panel size") relative to the traditional doctor's office.[21] *All without hiring more doctors.*

Who is going to see that early morning patient with the productive cough? Who is going to treat that dog bite at eight in the evening? Who is going to skip watching a great college football game to care for patients on that Saturday? The doctor whose patient population has grown by 20%, and whose office hours are now 6 days a week, 12 hours a day? No, *non-physicians* will join physicians in manning the PCMHs and providing care in other expanded service settings[22,23]; Primarily nurses,[24] physician and medical assistants, and some other allied health professionals. This is yet another reason that *these caregivers must now be considered providers.*

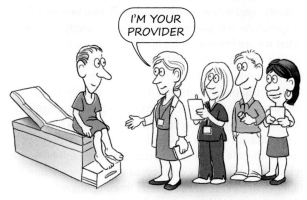

And sometimes we can't just stop with nurses, genetic counselors, allied health professionals and other "clinicians," because in many care scenarios, value-based patient-centered healthcare requires that our provider list travels to exotic places. A shuttle van driver may be a critical provider for a heart failure patient without other means of transportation to the pharmacy or doctor's office. A social worker may also be key to guiding a financially stressed stomach cancer patient in obtaining a costly chemotherapy drug directly from a pharmaceutical company at little or no cost. On a case-by-case basis, the provider team may include Case Managers, Patient Navigators, Insurance Specialists, Care Managers, Translators, Drivers, and many others who, prior to value-based reform, were viewed as peripheral players.

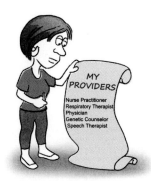

So a greatly expanded definition of THE PROVIDER is the first major change that we must accept and advance to successfully navigate our new healthcare system. *It now will take a team of providers working together to successfully deliver value-based care.* This concept is already manifesting as **interprofessional care** (the topic of an upcoming chapter), and it is one of the major movements pushing to achieve consistent, sustainable high value healthcare.

> *It now will take a team of providers working together to successfully deliver value-based care.*

So our definition of THE PROVIDER has been transformed from solo act to full ensemble. But do nurses, therapists, pharmacists, physician assistants, and all of the others who now populate the provider team now shoulder the same responsibilities that they had in the pre-reform, traditional healthcare system? Well, yes. While they must now be viewed as critical provider team members rather than as playing purely supportive roles, nurses and allied health professionals will continue to own their pre-reform responsibilities. And, *no.* Healthcare reform places additional responsibilities (often many) on allied health professionals, nurses, and others new to the official provider team.

For the most part, the new duties of the post-reform era fall into two major categories:

1. Clinical Knowledge and Skills
2. Business Knowledge and Acumen

For most nurses and allied health professionals, the changes in how we view and deliver healthcare will offer exciting opportunities to broaden their clinical knowledge and skills. As we previously noted, reform is shifting

PEARL

The replacement of our traditional fee-for-service reimbursement model with a payment based on value-based care dramatically redefines THE PROVIDER and provider responsibilities:

- The Doctor is no longer the sole provider. The new reform model demands that nurses, allied health professionals, and others are recognized members of the "provider" team.
- As providers, allied health professionals and nurses will have expanded clinical responsibilities, will need to broaden their business acumen, and may need to acquire new managerial skills.

healthcare to ambulatory settings, as we drive care towards the preventive and maintenance end of the care spectrum. This major transition in healthcare can only succeed if supported by our largest provider groups: nurses and allied health professionals. Clinical activities traditionally reserved for physicians (and in some cases, nurse practitioners) will more and more frequently fall to non-physicians, such as routine physical exams, chronic disease management, preventative screenings, patient education, and many, many more important care activities. In addition, clinical procedures traditionally performed by physicians and some nurse practitioners and physician assistants (e.g., wound care, skin biopsy, simple abscess drainage) may in the near future be performed by other "new providers." There is even active discussion about legalizing and training non-physicians to read x-rays and imaging studies, perform endoscopic screening exams, prescribe medications. Yes, truly today's healthcare reform represents *The Age of Nursing and Allied Health Professionals.*

> For most nurses and allied health professionals, the changes in how we view and deliver healthcare will offer exciting opportunities to broaden their clinical knowledge and skills.

But nurses and allied health professionals cannot focus on their new responsibilities within a clinical vacuum. *They must also gain and utilize new business knowledge and acumen.* Practices, hospitals, healthcare systems, ACOs, PCMHs, and all care organizations must now provide value-based care in order to be paid (again, in reality, to avoid damaging financial penalties). Therefore, *all providers* must deeply appreciate that in performing their clinical duties (both old and new), *they must view all of their care-related decisions through the lens of "value."* That means understanding both quality (the numerator in the value equation) and cost-efficiency (the denominator) when deciding on and providing patient care. Unnecessary tests must not be ordered (yes, a challenge in an environment of defensive medicine). Preventable errors must be avoided. *Failure to practice value-based care will not be a viable professional option.*

> All providers must deeply appreciate that in performing their clinical duties (both old and new), they must view all of their care-related decisions through the lens of "value."

In addition, some nurses and allied health professionals may need or choose to learn or improve their *managerial skills* if they wish to assume leadership roles in value-based care delivery organizations.

Of course, the big question is: *where will today's practicing nurses and allied health professionals initially and continuously gain the knowledge necessary to successfully fulfill these new clinical and business responsibilities?*

We'll get to that in a moment, under WHAT THE PROVIDER NEEDS. That said, much of the information and support that you'll have access to (likely available through your healthcare organization) will focus on the *clinical* aspects of your practice. Still, there's much that you can do right now as you seek to increase your business (and, should you need it, managerial), knowledge and skills. Continue to seek out information related to "the business of value-based healthcare." I say *continue,* because your reading this book is already for many of you the start of your value-based care educational journey. Search for courses, presentations, meetings, webinars, and publications aimed specifically at expanding your understanding of the business aspects of healthcare reform.

With that, let me just say, *welcome to the provider team!*

The Impact of Healthcare Reform on THE COIN OF THE REALM

In our traditional healthcare system, THE COIN OF THE REALM is money. In fact, this has not always been exactly true. Sometimes the doctor was paid in vegetables. In truth, the fee-for-service model preceded the US healthcare system by centuries. So whether the "Healer" received a Roman vase or the "Witchdoctor" was paid in live chickens, these were still monetary equivalents or "fees" to pay for "care services" rendered. Regardless of the form of payment, fee-for-service has rarely if ever linked the *outcome* of the provided "care" to the payment (ever hear of bloodletting?). No, the care provider was reimbursed with something of immediate, quantifiable value in exchange for "care" provided.

Now that our fast-paced healthcare delivery world is rapidly transitioning into value-based, preventive and maintenance care, money (and vegetables and chickens) have been replaced as THE COIN OF THE REALM. Because for today's numerous and varied providers, the most prized treasure amidst the daily chaos of clinical practice is not money.

It's *time.*

When healthcare *outcomes* are suddenly the focus of intense scrutiny, when the *quality of care* is closely

 PEARL

There is a new COIN OF THE REALM. Time has replaced money as the item most coveted by providers (money remains extremely important, but its attainment results from devoting time to consistently delivering high-value care).

evaluated, and when the *cost of care* is expressly analyzed, then *providers have to be more certain* when developing care plans and recommending care actions. And *it takes time* to be more certain that what you're recommending and doing does, in fact, represent "the best care." Often *significantly more time*. Now being "pretty sure" that a CT scan is the appropriate next step in evaluating Mrs. Murphy's abdominal pain carries financial risk (either directly or indirectly) for the provider. Now being "fairly certain" that Mr. Thomas doesn't need additional outpatient physical therapy carries financial risk for the provider. Now being "good" with simply watching that red blotch overlying Ms. Gordon's breast carries financial risk for the provider. The doctor, the nurse, the health professional, the hospital, the healthcare system… everyone affiliated with provider decisions is now at financial risk should those decisions be retrospectively categorized as of suboptimal value. So "pretty sure," "fairly certain," and "good" no longer cut it. Providers need to be more certain (often much more) that their care is of high value in terms of both quality and cost efficiency.

> *Providers have to be more certain* when developing care plans and recommending care actions. And *it takes time* to be more certain.

No, healthcare reform legislation doesn't penalize the physician assistant directly. The feds don't send treasury agents to the nurse's home to demand payment for sub-optimal delivered care. But healthcare reform legislation's more broadly defined "Provider," the hospital, healthcare system, ACO, or other care organization *which employs* the physician assistant, the nurse, and other individual providers, is penalized. And costing your employer organization money has a negative impact on resources, potentially worsening the quality of care that can be delivered. So in this indirect way, not spending adequate time to confirm the value of care decisions carries direct risk for the nurse, the health professional, and the doctor.

Where this really hits home is in *its impact on the practice of defensive medicine*. Remember that prior to reform, unless THE PROVIDER (The Doctor) was truly vexed in determining the next step in a patient's care, and unless a wrong choice was associated with significant patient risk, that physician would base care decisions on training, personal experience, and professional judgment. And if the physician was only "pretty sure" or "fairly certain" about a care recommendation or action, he or she would simply fall back on defensive medicine, ordering any and every test and procedure with a remote chance of helping to diagnose or treat the patient, wasting enormous amounts of money, potentially delaying appropriate care, and on rare occasion even placing the patient at risk (e.g., unnecessary biopsies). After all, *there were no reimbursement consequences for practicing defensive medicine.*

But no longer. Now both quality and cost-efficiency are retrospectively evaluated, analyzed, compared by outsiders, and both quality and cost-efficiency are directly linked to provider reimbursement. And now The Doctor is surrounded by many additional "providers." So now *every provider must consider all but the most routine care recommendations and actions in terms of quality and cost* because hospital readmission for a surgical wound infection in a patient who underwent an elective knee replacement is no longer an acceptable outcome; because a missed cervical cancer on routine pelvic exam is no longer an acceptable outcome; because failure to provide pneumonia vaccines to an elderly patient is no longer an acceptable outcome; and because delayed evaluation of a patient suffering a transient ischemic attack is no longer an acceptable outcome.

Because preventable medical errors are no longer acceptable.

There is already a list of legislated value-based reimbursement penalty programs threatening provider organizations, and this list expands annually (as do many of the penalty maximums). Thus, the financial risks facing providers are significant and increasing, and the need to get care "right the first time," both in terms of the quality and the cost efficiency, demands that today's providers *(including nurses and allied health professionals)* don't simply "go with their gut" when caring for their patients. Of course, the routine care that we all provide daily is of "the right care," right? Sure, the *rare patient* with the *uncommon disorder* will require providers to do a little research, but *not the average patient,* right?

Wrong.

Everywhere around the world that I travel (and that's a lot of places), I ask the providers the same one question: "Do your ICU patients get a chest x-ray every day?"

Invariably, they always answer "yes." (True, in China, one young, defensive physician said that their intensive care unit (ICU) patients receive chest x-rays every *other* day.)

Then I ask my follow-up question: "Why?"

This is always, *always* met with silence.

So I offer what I believe is the answer: "Because *that's what we've always done.* That's what we were all trained to do. That's what we all train our clinical students to do. Daily chest x-rays on ICU patients is *medical dogma.*"

Then I share the conclusions of an evidence-based study published by the American College of Radiology (an internationally recognized authority): "Routine daily chest radiograph in the ICU is not indicated."[25] I then show a slide that provides the study's evidence-based criteria for appropriate chest x-ray use in the ICU.

Finally, I conclude with a statement that makes them nod, but uncomfortably: "So, the evidence shows that for many if not most of our ICU patients, a routine, daily chest x-ray is of *no clinical benefit,* but it does unnecessarily deliver a daily dose of radiation to our patients' lungs and heart. And, of course, *it wastes a whole lot of money.*"

The cost of a portable chest x-ray in the United States varies widely, but suffice it to say that each study routinely costs several hundred dollars. Simply imagine the total cost of *thousands* of chest x-rays taken *daily* in ICUs across America. Think that money could be better spent elsewhere in our healthcare system? Say, *somewhere where it actually benefits patients?*

A humorous side note. That same, young, defensive Chinese physician who initially pushed back said, "Yes, many of our ICU chest x-rays are unnecessary. But while chest x-rays in the United States cost hundreds of dollars, here in China they cost the equivalent of, perhaps, forty American dollars."

"I understand your point," I replied. "And I have no reason to doubt that your ICU chest x-ray costs are much lower than ours." Then I remained silent for a moment before continuing. "That said, there are about 325 million Americans, and there are 1.4 *billion* Chinese. The United States has just over 5600 hospitals, while you have around *25,000*... in the end, I still respectfully suggest that you're wasting a large amount of money that could be better used elsewhere, and that the only thing many of your ICU patients are receiving is lung irradiation."

I must admit that I enjoyed seeing the subtle smile that flashed briefly across the lips of the senior Chinese physician sitting in the neighboring chair.

The point here is this: we don't just provide suboptimal care and waste money when caring for those *rare* patients suffering from *uncommon* diseases. *We provide suboptimal care and waste money every day in the routine care we provide our patients.*

Reflect on the *time implications* of this disturbing reality. Put it into a common analogy:

> Every morning you jump into your car. You start your car. You back out of your garage. You drive down streets, turning at corners, stopping at stop signs, merging into the adjacent lane. Braking. Accelerating. Checking your mirrors. Turning on your turn signal. Parking. Locking your car. *All without thinking.* Because you know how to do it, all of it, from the simple (putting your car in reverse) to the complex (merging at high speeds onto a crowded freeway).
>
> But what if you suddenly received a letter from your automobile insurance provider telling you that an entirely new model of insurance premium determination was being immediately implemented. Now your insurance premiums (that is, your insurance costs) will be directly based on how correctly and safely you perform every single driving decision and maneuver.
>
> You turned the key and started your car. Did you know that the engine specifications recommend you wait a certain period of time before first shifting out of park into reverse after first starting the engine? Too bad…your premium just went up.
>
> Forgot to flip on your turn signal indicator when turning left out of your driveway? Come on! It's your driveway! On your quiet little street! At 6 AM! Sorry… the law requires that you always indicate a planned turn, regardless of the driving location or environment. Up goes your premium again.
>
> Do you know how fast you were driving through the hospital parking lot? Eighteen miles per hour! *Where's the fire?!* After all, the posted speed limit within the lot is 15. Up, up, up your premium goes.

That's how it is in medicine today as reform sweeps across us like a flood. Recommendations, orders, decisions, procedures, blood tests, x-rays, biopsies, medications… many of the things that we do every day, *many of the things that we do without thinking* because we are confident that they are the right things to do for our patients, now come into question. Meaning that now before ordering that magnetic resonance imaging (MRI) study for that lower back pain, now before administering antibiotics for that cough, now before collecting a urine sample, *we must think about it.* And *thinking about what up to now has simply been automatic and routine is time consuming.*

> *We provide suboptimal care and waste money every day in the routine care we provide our patients.*

It takes time to search on-line, consult with a colleague, review a guideline. To find a credible source of current, "best practice" information. Not only to discover a high value approach in caring for your most challenging patients, but also to simply confirm that you are right when you are "pretty sure" or "fairly certain" of the next care move on a relatively routine case. And much like shoplifting, where the individual, minimal thefts accumulate into an enormous total sum of money lost, all of these little moments of additional stolen time (to confirm that you're providing appropriate care) add up, sucking precious minutes and quarter-hours out of each and every already overly busy day.

So the new COIN OF THE REALM in our new value-based world is *time.*

But don't just assume that with "time" replacing "money," providers aren't still extremely focused on getting paid. It's just that now time and money are intertwined, and protecting the former (time) is a constant battle for those providing patient care.

> Now time and money are intertwined, and protecting the former (time) is a constant battle for those providing patient care.

So we understand how healthcare reform has impacted THE PROVIDER and THE COIN OF THE REALM. Armed with this knowledge, we now move on to discuss the resulting big changes to the third major component of our healthcare system.

The Impact of Healthcare Reform on WHAT THE PROVIDER NEEDS

It used to be so simple. There was one provider (The Doctor), the healthcare model centered on one asset (money), and the one provider had only a few, simple needs (a Medical Degree and some books and journals).

My, *how things have changed.*

We've just discussed how the list of "providers" has grown, and how the responsibilities of all the now-numerous "providers" have greatly expanded with reform. And we've just reviewed how money (or chickens) has been surpassed by *time* as the most valuable provider asset. All of which leads to the question: *what do all of these varied providers need* to help them protect their valuable time while delivering high quality, cost-efficient patient care to ensure that they are paid?

There are several parts to the answer. Doctors, the traditional "providers," certainly need greater knowledge and skills in the age of healthcare reform. Not only is clinical information needed to keep up with direct "best care" trends, but so is new business (and often managerial) knowledge and skills. For example, a primary care physician running a Patient-Centered Medical Home is facing an entirely new world in terms of care delivery. That PCP's patient population has likely exploded to far larger than the traditional 1500-or-so patient panel. And likely the office is now open on Saturdays as well, perhaps from 7 AM until 9 at night. No longer employing two nurses and a receptionist to meet the expanded patient care population and schedule, the PCP now manages a rotating staff of five nurses, two physician assistants, and two receptionists.

And now, *the PCP no longer focuses exclusively on patient care.* Rather, the PCP now devotes a significant amount of time in activities that have only an indirect impact on the patients, such as supervising the clinical staff and administrative activities (for which many physicians are not trained). For many physicians, healthcare reform means at least participating in, and often overseeing, a more complex business, with far more non-physician staff caring for a larger patient population. Clearly, today doctors' needs are far broader and deeper (for some, *much broader and deeper*) than a Medical Degree and some books and journals gathering dust on a distant bookshelf...

But back to nurses and allied health professionals. In terms of WHAT THE PROVIDER NEEDS, there are three major categories:

1. Expanded Clinical Knowledge and Skills
2. Basic Business (and possibly Managerial) Knowledge and Skills
3. Expanded Educational Programs

The Expanded Clinical Needs of Nurse and Health Professional Providers

Let's go back to the example of the Patient-Centered Medical Home. New clinical responsibilities will suddenly be thrust upon the shoulders of the PCMH allied health professionals and nurses (the result of more patients and expanded office days and hours). Everything from routine physical exams, evaluation of common conditions, chronic disease care, screening… much of this will fall to non-physician providers. And as I mentioned, our new model of healthcare will likely push the boundaries of care responsibilities further (non-physicians reading x-rays, prescribing medications, performing endoscopy, etc.). No, I don't believe that shuttle van drivers will be performing open heart surgery, but I do believe that soon, nurses and health providers may well be performing some clinical duties that, up until now, they only watched physicians perform.

> New clinical responsibilities will suddenly be thrust upon the shoulders of the PCMH allied health professionals and nurses.

And that is exciting! After all, you entered healthcare to *care for patients.* Your timing couldn't have been more perfect. Healthcare reform is going to open many clinical doors to increased direct patient care responsibilities.

Exciting, yes. And *frightening.* Do you truly know how hard it is to accurately read a chest x-ray? You must examine every bone, the aorta, the heart, the pulmonary vasculature, the diaphragm, the lung parenchyma, the trachea, the mediastinum, the lymph nodes… all these shadows and more… for any subtle abnormality that might suggest disease. But we don't even have to consider such extreme potential responsibilities to understand the trepidation with which some providers may face new responsibilities.

On this Saturday evening, you're seeing a middle-aged man complaining of a sore throat. Your physical exam confirms a red, inflamed, irritated throat, and you take a swab to rapidly determine the presence of a *strep* infection. Not surprisingly, you also find soft, swollen, tender lymph nodes running down both sides of the patient's neck. And a single, swollen, lymph node just above his left clavicle (collar bone). All consistent with a pharyngitis.

Or is it? That supraclavicular lymph node is likely no different than the swollen, tender lymph nodes along the man's neck. Swollen and tender as a result of the patient's throat infection.

But…was that lone lymph node as tender as the others? And didn't it feel a little more firm?

The man has pharyngitis. But what if this one, slightly distant, slightly different-by-examination lymph node means that *he also has lymphoma?*

Should you order a CT scan of his chest? Should you arrange for a needle biopsy of this aberrant lymph node? Should you do nothing, simply wait and reexamine him (if he returns) in a few weeks?

Should you tell the patient of your concern? *Of your uncertainty?*

Remember, *value-based care is how the doctor, the staff, the entire practice get paid.* Doing the wrong thing (including doing nothing, if that's wrong) is a strike against value-based reimbursement. Doing too many things (ordering costly tests that prove unnecessary) is similarly a strike against value-based reimbursement.

Of course, you could just call the doctor, the PCP who is your partner and clinical supervisor and is still ultimately responsible for all patient care decisions. This is an appropriate, reasonable option. However, such care dilemmas are going to occur frequently (especially early on in our healthcare reform journey), so a doctor who is called throughout the day, sometimes at night, 6 days a week will soon burn out (and remember, time is THE COIN OF THE REALM for that doctor, too). Not to mention that you have your professional pride. *You want to do the right thing on your own,* based on your own knowledge and skill.

So, what do you need? What must the nurses and allied health professionals of today and tomorrow have to support "best care" practices?

Rapid access to easily usable expanded clinical knowledge and skills.

For the sake of our current discussion, let's talk about nurses and allied health professionals who have already completed their formal education and training and who are now actively practicing (either under the traditional healthcare system or in a new reform-based practice). You must continue caring for patients while also learning more about expanded (and often new) patient care activities. In other words, *you'll be fixing the airplane while the airplane is flying.*

You likely need help.

But take a breath… Help is available.

At the highest level, it's called **Clinical Decision Support (CDS).** There are many layers of CDS "solutions" (as these products and tools are broadly referred to). There are CDS solutions for nurses of all professional levels and for allied health professionals of virtually every stripe. And dozens and dozens of formats (text, video, images) and categories (reference solutions, skills, care plans, care pathways, order sets, drug information, etc.). Clinical Decision Support *is the key to empowering providers in consistently and sustainably delivering high value care.*

> Clinical Decision Support *is the key to empowering providers in consistently and sustainably delivering high value care.*

So do you want to learn more about CDS? Sorry… You'll have to wait until a little later in this book (Chapter 7 is devoted to CDS).

PEARL

Clinical Decision Support (explained in detail in Chapter 7) provides much of the value-based information needed for nurses and allied health professionals to succeed.

Basic Business (and Possibly Managerial) Knowledge and Skills

Some of the business and managerial knowledge and skills that nurses and allied health professionals need to successfully navigate healthcare reform are the same as those needed by physicians. Allied health professionals and nurses must possess *a basic understanding of value-based care.* Again, to your credit, you're already beginning (or continuing) your journey simply by picking up and (pretending to) learn from this book. And to truly appreciate value-based care, you'll need to better understand what lies at the heart of our new healthcare business model: *value-based reimbursement.*

It is estimated that *by 2018, as many as 90% of all Medicare payments will be value-based.*[26] Basically, that means that all of the healthcare you and your colleagues provide to Medicare patients will be reimbursed based on comparisons to government-defined quality and cost-of-care metrics.

> It is estimated that *by 2018, as many as 90% of all Medicare payments will be value-based.*

But *who are Medicare patients?*

Let's ask the federal government. According to the official Medicare website (Medicare.gov),[27] "Medicare is the federal health insurance program for people who are 65 or older, certain younger people with disabilities, and people with End-Stage Renal Disease..." There are several "Parts" to Medicare. "Medicare Part A" is "Hospital Insurance" and pays for care provided during hospitalizations, skilled nursing facility (SNF) stays, some types of home health visits, and end-of-life hospice. "Part B" is "Medical Insurance." This pays providers for certain physician services, ambulatory care services, specific medical supplies, and preventative care activities. Next comes "Part C," known as "Medicare Advantage Plans." This is a little more complicated. Medicare Advantage Plans are healthcare plans in which a private healthcare organization (and there are many types) has contracted with Medicare to cover the costs for all the benefits covered under Medicare Parts A and B. Finally, there is "Medicare Part D," better known as "Prescription Drug Coverage."

Now, not only is this more than you ever wanted to know about Medicare (unless you are currently covered by Medicare), but more than you need to know to practice value-based care. I'm sharing this synoptic overview of Medicare to make a point that you *do* need to understand and appreciate that *Medicare is a major payer in the American healthcare system.* According to The Kaiser Family Foundation, 17% of all Americans were covered by Medicare in 2015,[28] and the percentage of Medicare patients among those who seek care from healthcare providers is routinely much, much higher than that of the overall population. Think about it. *Older people* get sick. Relax... I understand that people younger than 65 break bones, suffer acute appendicitis, and get *strep* throat. Younger people even get cancer and other life-threatening illnesses. But older people routinely accumulate multiple health problems, have less physical reserve when faced with an acute exacerbation of a condition, and are often short on care assistance and general support. Thus, Medicare patients make up a large portion of America's inpatient (hospitalized patient) population. If you work in the inpatient setting, you understand what I'm saying here. In the last hospital in which I worked (a 300+ bed tertiary care center), more than 72% of our inpatients were Medicare beneficiaries. *72%.* Think this hospital is worried about value-based reimbursement? You bet.

Here's the point: with rare exception, very soon, *every provider will care for a large number of patients (likely the majority) whose care is reimbursed based on value.* Think about it. And if you're a *private health insurer,* and you see the federal government insurer (Medicare) projecting hundreds of millions of dollars or more in savings[29,30] by linking 90% or more of provider payments with quality and cost efficiency metrics defined by you, *what are you going to do?* You know the answer. The US government has not only legislated value-based reimbursement for federally insured patients, it has *legitimized value-based reimbursement for all patients, regardless of insurer.* There are piles of money to be salvaged here. Huge amounts of cash that private health insurers no longer feel required to dole out for the provision of lower value care outcomes, for care necessary to address preventable medical errors, and for the practice of defensive medicine.

> With rare exception, very soon, *every provider will care for a large number of patients (likely the majority of patients) whose care is reimbursed based on value.*

Value-based care, enforced via value-based reimbursement, will likely be adopted in some form by every insurer, both public and private. Sure, because it improves the quality of patient care, but let's be (cynically) honest: because it saves them money. The danger here, as I've previously suggested, is that in driving down costs, improved quality is not necessarily a certain consequence.

In the end, you must assume that value-based care is now the norm. In the previous section, we talked about the need for today's nurses and allied health professionals to expand their clinical skills and knowledge and how CDS solutions support that need. But with value improvement as our goal, CDS solutions must not only empower providers to deliver *high quality care.* CDS must be utilized by nurses and allied health professionals (along with doctors and other providers) to deliver *cost-efficient healthcare.* In other words, *clinical* providers must now demonstrate *business savvy* in care delivery. That means *understanding the financial implications of your care decisions and actions.*

> Sure, a urine culture would make absolutely certain that the antibiotic Melissa's provider will likely prescribe definitely covers the bacteria causing her bladder infection. Then again, Melissa is healthy. She's not pregnant. And she's had a urinary tract infection before. She even told her provider as soon as she entered the exam room, "I have a UTI." She has the classic history and symptoms. It is almost certain that her bladder infection is caused by a common bacteria, one that is covered by her provider's standard first-line antibiotic choice.

Melissa has a typical urinary tract infection that will respond to her provider's initial, standard prescribed antibiotic. No need to waste money on a urine culture.[31]

Today, some healthcare payers and providers aren't even waiting for the publication of peer-reviewed guidelines before challenging healthcare dogma. I recently learned of a very large, single-state healthcare system that had performed a retrospective analysis [unpublished] on the value of urinalysis in otherwise healthy, nonpregnant women presenting in the ambulatory setting with a classic history and symptoms typical of a urinary tract infection (UTI). Not on the value of *urine cultures*, mind you, but on the value of *urinalysis,* a standard practice nationwide. As in my previous tale of the unnecessary overuse of daily chest x-rays in ICUs across the world, this major healthcare system was questioning healthcare dogma, a care activity that seems engrained within our minds: must every healthy, nonpregnant woman "knows she has a UTI" have her urine analyzed for inflammatory cells and bacteria? What's the clinical benefit of all that cost? After all, now more than ever, providers must adopt the mantra: *"if it won't change your care, don't order it."*

Surprise, surprise. That major, multi-clinic healthcare system determined that the routine performance of urinalysis tests had failed to lead to a meaningful change in the initial antibiotic treatment for those women. Once again returning to our shoplifting example, while the cost of a single outpatient urinalysis was only $45, they were performing thousands and thousands of urinalysis tests annually, spending lots of money on tests that provided no benefit to their patients. Money that could be repurposed for other, beneficial healthcare purposes, reducing financial waste and driving down the cost-of-care across the system.

So even common tests and exams and procedures that you now or in the future will routinely order should on occasion be reevaluated, because some of what we all consider "standard of care" is likely either outdated or simply medical dogma, handed down from provider generation to provider generation without regular consideration or review. This doesn't mean that you have to memorize the cost of every blood test or understand the charge-to-payment ratio for every x-ray. It does mean, however, that you should understand *the most cost-efficient, clinically appropriate approach* to treating a routine urinary tract infection, community acquired pneumonia, sore throat, and other common conditions. You must learn to differentiate between the pain of gallstones and that of an acutely inflamed gallbladder (acute cholecystitis) through the most cost-efficient diagnostic pathway that ensures that if the diagnosis is the latter, you don't delay surgical treatment. You must appreciate that modifying your patient's dietary fiber is a less expensive initial approach to his intermittent constipation than a gastrointestinal motility study, and you must understand that while more cost-efficient, failing to order an endoscopic exam on a 63-year-old with rectal bleeding and visible hemorrhoids risks missing a rectal cancer. Thus, you must learn to *first identify the clinically appropriate pathway and then find a cost-efficient approach by which to travel that diagnostic and/or treatment path.*

> Thus, you must learn to *first identify the clinically appropriate pathway and then find a cost-efficient approach by which to travel that diagnostic and/ or treatment path.*

Quality of care can never be compromised to realize cost savings.

The evidence-based information available within CDS solutions can serve not only as your source of clinical information, but can also advance your business acumen. Many of today's (and future) clinical studies and trials directly address disease-specific costs-of-care, sharing insights on how to best financially manage patients without risking quality. Even information and guidance that does not specifically address costs still often represents "best practices," and deviating from such guidance should not be done without thoughtful consideration.

Most of the providers of today and tomorrow will not need to acquire additional managerial skills unless they will be serving in administrative and/or practice leadership roles (as in the case of providers serving in leadership roles within PCMHs or ACOs). Thus, while many of us will need expanded clinical and business knowledge and skills, only a minority will also need advanced managerial skills. But for this cohort, those who choose roles in which others fall under their supervision, learning how to support, educate, empower, discipline—*learning how to manage*—will be critical to achieving professional success and realizing personal satisfaction. When it comes to *managerial* skills, most of today's CDS solutions are of limited value. Managerial courses, human resources workshops, and other targeted training programs, however, are of great value. Most are designed to fit into the workflow of the busy healthcare provider (such as webinars and 1- or 2-day seminars). I encourage any of you who will serve in or might consider such leadership positions to seek out such targeted training opportunities.

The Expanded Educational Needs of Nurse and Health Professional Students

Let's take a moment and think about the nurses and allied health professionals of *tomorrow*. That is, students who must be educated and trained not only to function, but to *succeed* once they matriculate into a healthcare system in which they are no longer viewed as "physician extenders" but as true "providers," a system in which they will have greater clinical responsibilities than previous graduates. In which every aspect of the care they provide must be value-based.

The titanic shift in our healthcare environment represents enormous challenges for our educational institutions, whether public or private. It seems doubtful that many of today's nursing and/or health professional educational institutions currently have the appropriate staff, tools, and/or finances necessary to train today's students to meet the new challenges resulting from the healthcare reform of today and tomorrow.

> The titanic shift in our healthcare environment represents enormous challenges for our educational institutions.

But here, too, CDS solutions are already providing much of what our educational institutions and future-providers need. There are CDS solutions specifically designed to empower nurses and health educators in identifying strengths and weaknesses in their individual student's knowledge base and skills. Other CDS solutions allow teachers to rapidly and efficiently organize current, credible information (including videos, skills training, high definition graphics, peer-reviewed articles, etc.) into lessons and student study guides. And for students, new, multiple-format CDS solutions are available to educate the provider-in-training on a variety of clinical topics and skills. And here's an additional significant benefit: students who have utilized CDS solutions throughout their training will no doubt be at least fairly comfortable in continuing use of CDS solutions in patient care following graduation.

For the near term, educational institutions will need to continually modify their curricula to meet their students' new clinical and business knowledge and skills needs. Schools will have to hire new staff, individuals with the knowledge

PEARL

Providers now need expanded clinical knowledge and skills, basic business knowledge and skills, and (for some) managerial skills. Educational institutions must rapidly adopt new curricula and hire additional, experienced faculty to address similar additional areas of educational needs for their students.

and experience to teach our students what they need to learn how to successfully practice in our new healthcare world. Of course, all of this (CDS solutions, additional staff and resources) costs money. As is the case for many hospitals and healthcare systems today, many educational institutions face the challenge of currently being financially strapped while needing additional investments to provide their students what they need to succeed.

Summary

You now understand that you are no longer on the outside. You are no longer a "physician extender." You, too, are THE PROVIDER. You now or will likely soon have expanded clinical responsibilities and opportunities. Indeed, *it is an exciting time to be an allied health or nurse provider!*

You also now appreciate that while money is (of course) very important to you, to the other providers with whom you work, to your practice, and to your employer, the new COIN OF THE REALM is *time*, because some of the care that you have always provided without a second thought may now need…a second thought. Now both the quality and the cost of your care will be retrospectively scrutinized to determine whether the *value* (quality/cost) of your care was appropriate.

Those of you already practicing in the real world may need considerable help in stepping up to true value-based care. You need rapidly accessible, easily usable, workflow-friendly, current, credible, evidence-based information, knowledge, and guidance (that's a mouthful, but that's today's healthcare). You need to understand the implications of your care recommendations and actions in terms of both quality and cost. Fortunately, much of what you need is available in the form of CDS solutions. (Again, Chapter 7 is focused on CDS.) For those interested in a managerial role (as the number and responsibilities of such positions are increasing), you'll need sources of information other than CDS to advance your knowledge and skillset. Fortunately, this is a growing cottage industry, as there is money to be made by providing expert managerial training to healthcare providers.

Finally, our educational institutions face several major challenges. Students must gain additional clinical knowledge and attain new clinical skills. However, their education must not be limited to the clinical aspects of care alone. Now nurses and allied health professionals must understand the business basics of value-based healthcare. They must become facile in the real-time use of CDS solutions to guarantee not only the clinical quality, but also the cost-efficiency of the care they will be providing. They must be taught not only how to function, not only how to survive, but also *how to lead in this new healthcare world.* These are enormous educational demands. In response, our health professional training programs and nursing schools must rapidly expand and modify their curricula to ensure that their students are successful once having graduated into the new healthcare environment.

References

1. Porter ME. What is value in health care? *N Engl J Med.* 2010;363:2477–2481.
2. Zuvekas SH, Cohen JW. Paying physicians by capitation: is the past now prologue? *Health Aff.* 2010;29:1661–1666.
3. *CMS: The 2,225 Hospitals that Will Pay Readmissions Penalties Next Year.* The Advisory Board (online); 2013. https://www.advisory.com/daily-briefing/2013/08/05/cms-2225-hospitals-will-pay-readmissions-penalties-next-year.
4. Satran J. *Is Obamacare Punishing Hospitals the Wrong Way?* The Huffington Post (online); 2015. http://www.huffingtonpost.com/entry/obamacare-hospital-readmissions_us_55f732e1e4b0c2077efbb909.
5. Serrie J. *More than 2,200 Hospitals Face Penalties Under ObamaCare Rules.* Fox News (online); 2012. http://www.foxnews.com/politics/2012/08/23/more-than-2200-hospitals-face-penalties-for-high-readmissions.html.
6. Rau J. *Nearly 1,500 Hospitals Penalized Under Medicare Program Rating Quality.* Kaiser Health News (online); 2013. http://khn.org/news/value-based-purchasing-medicare/.
7. Rice S. *Most Hospitals Face 30-Day Readmissions Penalty in Fiscal 2016.* Modern Healthcare (online); 2015. http://www.modernhealthcare.com/article/20150803/NEWS/150809981.
8. *The State of Hospitals' Financial Health.* American Hospital Association: Advancing Health in America (online); 2002. http://www.aha.org/content/00-10/Wp2002HospFinances.pdf.
9. Evans M. *Hospitals Face Closures as 'A New Day in Healthcare' Dawns.* Modern Healthcare (online); 2015. http://www.modernhealthcare.com/article/20150221/MAGAZINE/302219988.
10. Kutscher B, Evans M. *The New Normal?* Modern Healthcare (online); 2013. http://www.modernhealthcare.com/article/20130810/MAGAZINE/308109974.
11. Zaino J. *Changing Priorities Shift Hospital Focus to Outpatient Strategies.* Healthcare Finance (online); 2014. http://www.healthcarefinancenews.com/news/changing-priorities-shift-hospital-focus-outpatient-strategies.
12. Young J. *Why We're Picking Walmart and CVS Over Doctors' Offices.* The Huffington Post (online); 2015. http://www.huffingtonpost.com/2015/01/12/retail-clinics_n_6445506.html.

13. Resnick J. *Bring Health Care Home*. The New York Times (online); 2011. http://www.nytimes.com/2011/12/05/opinion/bring-health-care-home.html.

14. Naylor M, Keating SA. Transitional Care: Moving Patients from One Care Setting to Another. *Am J Nurs*. 2008;108:58–63.

15. Ross C. *New Trends Moving Healthcare to the Home*. Mindflow Design (online); 2016. http://www.mindflowdesign.com/insights/new-trends-moving-healthcare-to-the-home/.

16. Burke A. *DNA Sequencing Is Now Improving Faster Than Moore's Law!* Forbes (online); 2012. https://www.forbes.com/sites/techonomy/2012/01/12/dna-sequencing-is-now-improving-faster-than-moores-law/#3d2a3ec45e4f.

17. U.S. Department of Labor, Bureau of Labor Statistics (online) 2015; https://www.bls.gov/ooh/healthcare/genetic-counselors.htm.

18. National Society of Genetic Counselors (online) 2017; http://www.nsgc.org/page/aboutgeneticcounselors.

19. Adler EL. *Practices Considering PCMH Model Must Consider Challenges*. Physicians Practice (online); 2013. http://www.physicianspractice.com/blog/practices-considering-pcmh-model-must-consider-challenges.

20. Patient Centered Medical Home Resource Center. Department of Health and Human Services: AHRQ (online); https://pcmh.ahrq.gov/page/defining-pcmh.

21. Berra A. *PCMH Panel Size Trends: Introducing a New Data Series*. Advisory Board: The Blueprint (online); 2012. https://www.advisory.com/research/health-care-advisory-board/blogs/the-blueprint/2012/05/examining-pcmh-panel-size-trends.

22. *NPP Utilization in the Future of US Healthcare*. Medical Group Management Association (online); 2014. https://www.mgma.com/Libraries/Assets/Practice%20Resources/NPPsFutureHealthcare-final.pdf.

23. *Physician Assistants and the Patient-Centered Medical Home*. American Academy of Physician Assistants: Professional Issues (online); 2011. http://www.mainepa.com/pdf/PI_PAs_PCMH_Final.pdf.

24. *New Approaches for Delivering Primary Care Could Reduce Predicted Physician Shortage*. Rand Corporation (online); 2013. http://www.rand.org/content/dam/rand/pubs/research_briefs/RB9700/RB9752/RAND_RB9752.pdf.

25. Amrosa JK, Bramwit MP, Mohammed TL, et al. ACR appropriateness criteria: routine chest radiographs in intensive care unit patients. *J Ame Coll Rad*. 2013;10:170–174.

26. *90% of Medicare Will Be Value-Based Reimbursement by 2018*. HealthIT Analytics (online); 2015. http://healthitanalytics.com/news/90-of-medicare-will-be-value-based-reimbursement-by-2018.

27. What's Medicare? Medicare.gov (online); https://www.medicare.gov/sign-up-change-plans/decide-how-to-get-medicare/whats-medicare/what-is-medicare.html.

28. *Medicare Beneficiaries as a Percent of Total Population*. Henry J. Kaiser Family Foundation (online); 2015. http://kff.org/medicare/state-indicator/medicare-beneficiaries-as-of-total-pop/?currentTimeframe=0&sortModel=%7B%22colId%22:%22Location%22,%22sort%22:%22asc%22%7D.

29. Mangan D. Obamacare Program Generates 'Substantial' Medicare Savings. *CNBC (online)*. 2015;. http://www.cnbc.com/2015/05/04/obamacare-program-generates-substantial-medicare-savings.html.

30. Amadeo K. *CBO Report on Obamacare Costs, Savings and Impact on Economy*. The Balance (online); 2016. https://www.thebalance.com/cbo-report-obamacare-3305627.

31. *Treatment of Urinary Tract Infections in Nonpregnant Women*. American College of Obstetricians and Gynecologists; 2008 . Practice Bulletin:10.

CHAPTER 5

The Map to Get There: The Triple Aim

I remember explaining to my youngest daughter how her mother and I grew up in a world without Snapchat, without Amazon, without Google, without the internet. And without a global positioning system (GPS).

"Daddy," she said, a concerned look crossing her face, "if there was no GPS, did you and Mommy ever go out?"

Hiding my amusement as best as I could, I replied. "Well, yes, Honey. Mommy and I would climb onto our dinosaur and head out to McDonalds." Then I added, "But of course, we often got lost."

We know where we want to go: we want to cure cancer; to end world hunger; we want peace in the Middle East. Selecting our "destinations" is often the easy part. It's developing, implementing, and following a path to successfully arrive at those destinations that routinely poses the greatest challenges. So it is that in seeking meaningful healthcare reform, we need a clear, understandable, and powerful roadmap.

The Triple Aim

Fortunately, we have one; or at least, the US government (and, subsequently, the nation's private health insurers) has found one. It's called *The Triple Aim,*[1] and it has been enthusiastically adopted by the federal government to serve as our healthcare GPS. The Triple Aim, as the name implies, has three components that together are intended to direct us down the path to meaningful, value-based patient care. Developed and promoted by the **Institute for Healthcare Improvement (IHI),** a highly respected, internationally recognized healthcare think-tank, The Triple Aim has now been widely adopted to serve as "a framework… that describes an approach to optimizing health system performance.[1]"

Understanding The Triple Aim, like understanding the instructions voiced by your car's GPS, is essential for anyone working in healthcare today. So let's explore The Triple Aim.

> ● **PEARL**
>
> The Triple Aim has been adopted by the government, private payers, and most healthcare organizations as our "GPS roadmap" to successful reform.

Aim #1: Improving the Patient Experience of Care

Perhaps no healthcare reform concept is more truly disruptive than the first component of The Triple Aim: "Improving the **patient experience** of care (including quality and satisfaction)."

Improving *the patient experience?* What is this, *Disney World?*

Yes.

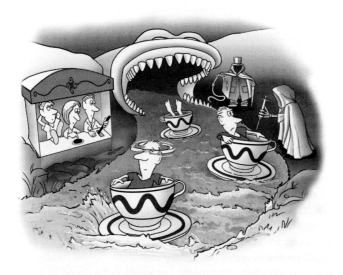

It's not an accident that the name "Disney" is synonymous with "great family experience." Mothers and fathers don't just randomly select Disney World as the recipient of their valuable time and financial resources. We select theme parks, vacation sites, restaurants, clothing…practically everything for which we have a choice whether to buy, visit, or utilize based on the projected favorability of the experience: the *quality* of the experience versus the *cost* (that is, the *value* of the opportunity). It is in this, the first component of The Triple Aim, that another true revolutionary principle of today's healthcare reform is demonstrated. No longer is healthcare defined by, regulated through, and focused so heavily on the traditional provider, the doctor; the reins are now being handed over to *the patient.* Now *the patient's experiences* during interactions with the healthcare system are a critical factor in the assessment of the value of delivered care.[2]

So thoroughly did the federal government accept and adopt this IHI roadmap to US healthcare reform that today, *a significant minority of provider organization reimbursement is dependent on evidence of a favorable patient experience.*[3] In other words, *if patients have a poor experience, providers lose money.* And how do payers assess "the patient experience?" For inpatients, through a multiple question survey called **HCAHPS, the Hospital Consumer Assessment of Healthcare Providers and Systems.**[4–6] (For patients receiving care in hospital outpatient departments or from ambulatory surgery centers, the Centers for Medicare and Medicaid is now implementing **OAS CAHPS, the Outpatient and Ambulatory Surgery Consumer Assessment of Healthcare Providers and Systems.**[7])

> *A significant minority of provider organization reimbursement is dependent on evidence of a favorable patient experience.* In other words, *if patients have a poor experience, providers lose money.*

The HCAHPS survey is designed to capture data that then allows for uniform comparisons across hospitals of adult inpatients' satisfaction regarding their recent hospitalizations. Not surprisingly, many survey questions focus directly on medical care issues, such as "nurse communication," "physician communication," "pain management," and "communication about medicines." Other questions, however, are nonmedical, assessing *care activities,* such as "staff responsiveness" and "care transitions." And finally, there are questions that might just as likely be found in a

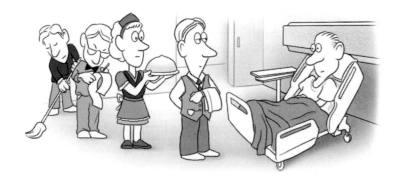

survey of recent hotel guests such as rating the "cleanliness" and "quietness" of the "hospital environment."

So reform links the quality and cost of care to provider reimbursement and some of that quality is determined by "the patient experience." This sudden focus on how the patient views and feels about his or her time in the hospital has led to the explosive growth in Patient Experience from cottage industry to major healthcare sector focus. New varieties of hospital leaders have burst onto the healthcare scene, carrying titles such as "Director of Patient Experience" and "Patient Experience Intelligence Officer." Even the word "patient" has been replaced in many facilities and systems, with hospitalized individuals now often referred to as "customers,"[8] "clients," "consumers,"[9] or "guests." At first, this dramatic shift from seemingly objective, medically focused hospitals to consumer-friendly "hospital environments" tends to make many providers roll their eyes. However, the deeper purpose of this new approach will hopefully ultimately achieve for healthcare what is successfully achieved every day across thousands of markets and industries: *drive value improvement.* Healthcare is finally at least dipping its toe into the world of dining, of car sales, and of apartment rentals; that is, *factoring in consumer preference.* Websites offering assessments and evaluations of individual doctors and hospitals have sprung up all over the web, and regardless of accuracy or credibility (a separate but important topic), patients now have access to information that they can use in making choices about where and from whom they receive care.

> Patients now have access to information that they can use in making choices about where and from whom they receive care.

Still, most of the information available online today fails to address the non-medical care metrics measured by some of the HCAHPS survey questions; rather, most online comparison and review sites offer consumers data on relatively objective clinical metrics, such as infection and complication rates and treatment-specific days of hospitalization. At present, then, it's much like a restaurant review that only offers an assessment of the food, failing to compare or review the wait for a table, the atmosphere, or the service.

"How was your dinner?" I asked my friend, expectantly. A new restaurant had opened in our small town. Given that the neighborhood pizzeria was considered the pinnacle in local dining, I was eager to hear his tale of exotic appetizers, glorious dishes, and enticing bar drinks, all offered by the much-anticipated "high-end" restaurant that had finally opened its doors in our little community.

"Well," he said, his tone one of obvious disappointment, "it was OK." He paused and then added, "I mean, the food was great. Really exceptional."

But it was obvious that his overall impression was one of mediocrity. I waited in silence for the explanation, which soon followed.

"The whole place is just one big room. And there's no carpeting or plants or anything to dull the noise. It was so loud that we couldn't hear each other speak across the table."

Hmmm… lousy dining environment.

"And the waiter was so rushed, so stressed. They had way too few waiters and waitresses, so it made the whole experience feel a bit anxious."

Hmmm… rushed, stressed-out staff.

"But still, the food was good."

"Are you going back?" I asked, curious as to which way his scale would tip.

He thought for a moment. "Well," he finally concluded, "only if they make it quieter, and if they get more wait-staff. I mean, the food's great, but it costs way too much to have an unhappy waiter and so much noise you can't hear your friends."

The fact is, while good food is central to the dining experience (in the absence of good food, no amount of atmosphere and congenial staff is likely to result in return customers), there are many additional factors that contribute to diner satisfaction. In this regard, the actual medical care provided by physicians, nurses, and allied health professionals is loosely analogous to the restaurant food. Yes, having a nurse who demonstrates the competence and skills to care for a postoperative patient is critical to the patient's overall clinical outcome; however, competence and skills alone do not guarantee a positive patient experience. It's similar to that common question, "Would your rather have a surgeon with a great bedside manner or a surgeon with great surgical skills?" Prior to reform, the standard answer was, "great surgical skills." In today's healthcare world, the answer is: *the patient expects both.*

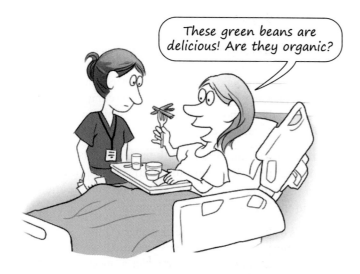

The Triple Aim demands high-quality patient care, where quality includes not only the patient's objective clinical outcome, but also the patient's subjective experience regarding the caregivers, caregiver activities, and the care environment. So which providers are most influential in creating a favorable patient experience? The truth is, and the questions comprising the HCAHPS survey reflects this (more questions which relate to nurses and "hospital staff"), that only limited actual activities impacting the patient experience fall to the physician. Physicians as a group (and surgeons and other proceduralists more specifically) spend very little time directly interacting with their patients relative to the time provided by nurses, allied health professionals, and many other hospital staff. (Even physician ambulatory visits tend to be relatively brief.) Thus, the physician needs to be communicative and at least somewhat pleasant to avoid a negative rating on the few HCAHPS physician-related survey questions. On the other hand, the care provided by nurses, allied health professionals, by transportation and food preparation and food delivery, and janitorial and other "hospital staff" can significantly impact HCAHPS scores.

It may surprise you, but healthcare facility and system *administrators* play a significant role in assuring positive experiences for their patients, through the allocation of resources (both human and financial). But it is *nurses and allied health professionals who offer the greatest opportunity to succeed (or fail) in providing a favorable experience to our patients and their loved ones.* After all, no provider spends nearly the amount of time that nurses (in particular) and allied health professionals allocate to interacting with patients and patient families. Nor does any other healthcare professional provide the breadth of care offered by nurses whose responsibilities range from the purely clinical (medications administration, wound care, etc.) to the personal (comforting those in pain and distress, providing counseling and advice, etc., etc.) to the important but mundane (daily weights, provision of bedpans, etc., etc., etc.).

> It is nurses and allied health professionals who offer the greatest opportunity to succeed (or fail) in providing a favorable experience to our patients and their loved ones.

Let's be honest here. In the past, physicians, administrators, and even patients regarded many of the numerous and varied nursing activities as niceties, but of limited importance in the overall picture of "healthcare." But just take a look at the HCAHPS survey questions (which you can easily find online)[10] and you'll see how dramatically that previous, traditional healthcare views have changed. With the first component of The Triple Aim, with the direct impact of "the patient experience" on payments to hospitals and healthcare systems, our view of nurses and nursing activities has been flipped on its head. Now these once "niceties" have edged up just behind a nurse's clinical duties in terms of importance (from a reimbursement perspective). Sure, making certain to administer the correct insulin dose via the correct route at the correct time is critical, but allowing a hemodynamically stable patient to sleep through the night undisturbed (if appropriate, based on clinical status and scenario), or immediately responding to a call light are now also important not just to the patient, but to the entire provider team and organization.

The nurse who is warm, caring, attentive… who listens, touches, shares… has a dramatic, favorable effect on the experience of the patient and that of the patient's family and friends (as well as on other clinical staff). This is where healthcare administrators must step up, because with the tightening of resources, nurses and allied health professionals are often finding themselves with less and less time per patient and more and more to do per patient. The result? A less engaged, more stressed care provider, leading to potentially poorer patient care and a poorer experience for the patient[11] (remember the impact of the stressed-out waiter on my friend's dining experience?). So with patient experience now directly linked to reimbursement, hospital and outpatient facility administrators would be wise to consider (and nurses, allied health professionals, and other staff to aggressively point out) the need to allocate adequate human and financial resources to ensure that all providers are truly able to treat their "guests" appropriately.

In today's world of healthcare reform, nurses are the foot soldiers in the drive to achieve the first component of The Triple Aim: Improving the Patient Experience of Care.

Aim #2: Improving the Health of Populations

Prior to the recent tectonic shift in our thinking, you could have asked virtually any one (patient, therapist, physician, nurse, payer) to define "healthcare" and you would have received some version of the same response: *"the doctor-patient relationship."* The doctor-patient relationship is a term burned into the American lexicon. For centuries, the doctor-patient relationship has not only been at the heart of healthcare, it has for all intents and purposes been *the definition of healthcare.*

But no longer.

Defining healthcare as "the doctor-patient relationship" is no longer viable, not in our nation, where greater than 17% of our country's gross domestic product is spent providing healthcare of overall mediocre quality (or worse); not in China (the most populous country on earth), where Alzheimer disease already affects more than 9 million but where only a handful of dementia experts practice[12,13]; not in Brazil's Amazon region,[14] where cervical cancer is the leading cause of cancer deaths among women despite the availability of preventative vaccines. The truth is that a model so narrowly focused (as well as so asymmetrically focused on one member of the pair, the doctor) clearly cannot keep the world's healthcare systems from plunging into the abyss.

> For centuries, "the doctor-patient relationship" has not only been at the heart of healthcare, it has for all intents and purposes been *the definition of healthcare.* But no longer.

Enter *Population Health Management* (also simply referred to as **Population Health**). Known by the acronym **PHM,** this new view of health and healthcare represents a 180-degree U-turn from the traditional focus of healthcare on the doctor-patient relationship. Instead of considering how Dr. Smith treats his diabetics, PHM directs us to consider *the patient* at the center of healthcare. But PHM strays even further from our traditional concept of healthcare in refusing to individualize Mr. Jones as a type 2 diabetes patient and then Mrs. Smith as a different type 2 diabetes patient (as if they were apples and oranges); rather, PHM asks us to consider *both Mr. Jones and Mrs. Smith together,* as part of a larger pool of individuals who all share the risks and needs of type 2 diabetes sufferers. That is, Mr. Jones and Mrs. Smith are *part of a specific patient population.* A population with unique and clear educational, prevention, care, and treatment needs and *care opportunities.*

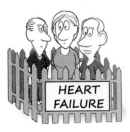 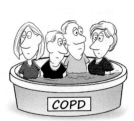 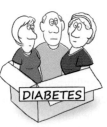

The definition of a PHM population also does not need to be based on a *clinical condition.* For example, a population defined as "Emergency Room Frequent Fliers" (patients who visit their emergency room significantly more frequently than the average patient) may well offer clear opportunities to improve care, resulting in reduced ER usage and costs and a better quality of life for the targeted patient population. Perhaps the Frequent Fliers lack access to primary care or have failed to take their prescription medications. Alternatively, you could define a population as all females of appropriate age who have failed to undergo their recommended mammogram screening or cancer patients unable to afford their chemotherapy copayments.

Thus, *the definition of a PHM population is fluid.* The *goal* of PHM, however, *is not.* PHM seeks to *define populations for which common interventions (educational, medical, social, logistical, etc.) can improve health and reduce the costs of care.*

Two town mayors find themselves next to one another on the banks of a river.

"My townspeople are starving," says the first, as he casts his line out into the flowing waters. "I'm going to try and catch fish after fish after fish in hopes of feeding them."

"My townspeople are starving as well," replies the second. Then, he casts a large net into the river, capturing an entire school of fish.

Our populations around the world, and our nations and economies, are starving for higher value healthcare. "The doctor-patient relationship" is the town mayor with the single fishing pole who hopes to catch one fish at a time. "Population Health" is… well, you get it.

Population Health Management seeks to define populations for which common interventions (educational, medical, social, logistical, etc.) can improve health and reduce the costs of care.

So, *who will drive PHM programs?*

The answer, like many answers to the questions engendered by healthcare reform, is a variety of providers *(including patients).* Certainly, physicians play a role from identifying and defining target populations offering interventional opportunities to strategizing and implementing interventional activities and to assessing intervention efficacy and driving tactical modifications. But once again, *it's nurses and allied health professionals who must play key roles* if these defined populations (which include our families, our friends, our neighbors, our fellow citizens) are to realize better health and if our economies and wallets are to realize financial relief. PHM demands that inpatient and ambulatory pharmacists, nurses, therapists, dieticians, technologists, other allied health professionals, as well as healthcare administrators, and (yes!) patients join physicians in *shedding the mantra that the "doctor-patient relationship" is the definition of healthcare.* And we must all *broaden our view of patients as only individuals in need of healthcare.* Providers must now look to identify characteristics from which *populations of patients* can be defined to improve the quality and cost of their care from not only obvious, condition-based cohorts (such as "Heart Failure Patients" or "COPD Patients"), but also individuals who share socio-economic-demographic characteristics that may be impeding high value care delivery (such as those patients without transportation or those who are too financially stressed to seek care). As we are seeing time and time again with reform activities, *it is nurses and allied health professionals who must serve as the cornerstone of population health management.* Who better than these providers who routinely spend more time with patients than physicians and who regularly best "know the patients and their families" to help identify such populations and participate in the development, implementation, and refinement of population health improvement programs and processes?

As we concluded for the first Aim, nurses and allied health professionals will determine the success in our push to achieve Aim #2.

> ● **PEARL**
>
> Aim #2 defines a major shift from "the doctor-patient relationship" to Population Health Management as the focus of healthcare activities.

Aim #3: Reducing the Per Capita Cost of Healthcare

At first glance, the third goal of The Triple Aim appears to be in direct conflict with Aim #2 (Population Health Management). After all, the very words "per capita" mean *"by or for each individual person."*[15] So how can a hospital, let alone a society, achieve the seemingly conflicting goals of both improving the health of *populations* while simultaneously focusing on each *individual* patient?

Harken back to a simpler time when the most advanced form of communication was a telephone… attached to a wall… by a cord. When you *had to watch* television commercials. When in many rooms, and certainly in the den, there were *bookshelves.* A long row of dusty, earth-tone volumes standing upright or leaning at gentle angles, the line of tomes running horizontally across the shelf. And holding that vast collection of printed knowledge in place? *Bookends.* One on each side the row of books. Two bookends, seemingly in constant battle, pushing in direct opposition to one another; but in reality, *needing each other* to achieve the required equilibrium lest the books topple to the floor.

All right… let me pull back from my romantic reflections. I know… bookends are rarely seen today, as bookshelves have largely been replaced by wireless tablets and smartphones. That said, the analogy is apt. *The dual goals of population health management and per capita healthcare cost reduction are bookends.* Not only are they *not* mutually exclusive, together they can define a delicate equilibrium that allows us to achieve greater health and healthcare value.

> *The dual goals of population health management and per capita healthcare cost reduction are bookends.*

Let's return to dear Mr. Jones and sweet Mrs. Smith, both of whom you will recall suffer from type 2 diabetes. Considering these two individuals as members of a larger pool of patients in our *Type 2 Diabetes Population Health Management Program* is a reasonable, even obvious strategy. Their providers or hospital (or insurer) may be attempting to improve the quality of health for all of their type 2 diabetic patients through patient education and early interventional care. And not only will reducing cardiovascular events, decreasing renal failure, and performing fewer leg amputations benefit the patients in terms of *quality,* such PHM will also benefit everyone in terms of overall (and per capita) reductions in the *cost* of care for this population of type 2 diabetics.

But there's even more we can learn in considering the population-versus-individual healthcare model. Whether intentional or not, the "per capita" of Aim #3 makes broader implications for the population goal of Aim #2. We must appreciate that the danger in seeking to improve health and healthcare only (or most heavily) on the *population* level is analogous to depending only (or most heavily) on one bookend to keep our books perched safely upright on the shelf. Because while Mr. Jones and Mrs. Smith do indeed share a common, medically significant diagnosis (type 2 diabetes), they are also *medically and socio-economic-demographically unique individuals.* Perhaps Mr. Jones has already experienced a heart attack and now suffers from mild congestive heart failure. He lives alone, has no car, and survives on the little he receives in Social Security benefits. Mrs. Smith is already struggling with lower extremity diabetic neuropathy and vascular impairment, resulting in her already having suffered from diabetic foot ulcers and the constant risk of future amputation. She lives with her daughter's family in an affluent section of town. Mr. Jones and Mrs. Smith are simultaneously similar (both type 2 diabetics) and dissimilar, in terms of the clinical courses of their diabetes, their support network, and their financial capabilities.

> The danger in seeking to improve health and healthcare only (or most heavily) on the *population* level is analogous to depending only (or most heavily) on one bookend to keep your books perched safely upright on the shelf.

OK, so Mr. Jones and Mrs. Smith are similar and dissimilar. How does that help?

It helps because in focusing us on the patient as an individual, Aim #3 further empowers Aim #2, Improving the Health of Populations. That is, *the more we understand our patients as individuals, the more effective we can be in caring for our patients within populations.*

> Think about your son or daughter. A pure population perspective means that your school views your child only as a "Third Grader." The fact is, your kid is exceptionally strong in math but struggles a little bit with reading. If the third grade teacher gets to know each child as an individual, the population of "Third Graders" can be further divided into populations to the benefit of the children. Your child will flourish as part of the population of third-graders taught math at an accelerated rate, and your child will likewise benefit from also being viewed as a member of the third grade population who receives a little extra help to improve reading skills. This is population management resulting from individualization. Fortunately for our children (and our society), the bookends of individualization and population-based teaching are routinely used to maximize the value of our educational processes.

There's an important difference between your third-grader and most patients. While your child's individual characteristics place him or her in one math population and in another reading population, in healthcare, our populations' defining characteristics need to be more complex if we are to truly improve value. While your child benefits from being in one math population and a second reading population, it may be far less valuable for Mr. Jones, his providers, and those paying for his care to include him in one Type 2 Diabetes PHM program and a different Heart Failure Patients PHM program. Wouldn't it be better (both in terms of quality and cost) if Mr. Jones is a member of a single PHM program that seeks to improve the health of type 2 diabetics with heart failure? After all, it's not a small group.[16]

Why would this be better?

There are many causes of heart failure, and those underlying etiologies have *different implications for patient care.* Mr. Jones' heart failure is the result of his type 2 diabetes (courtesy of a myocardial infarction). Including Mr. Jones in a population of *all* patients with heart failure, many of whose cardiac disease *did not result from type 2 diabetes,* would be less useful than implementing a more etiology-specific stratification process. Mr. Jones, his providers, and Medicare (that's all taxpayers) will likely achieve greater value if he is included in a PHM program targeting "Type 2 Diabetics With Heart Failure." In fact, there may be even greater value in a PHM program for "Type 2 Diabetics With Heart Failure and Who Are Without Transportation and Have Limited Financial Resources." I may be getting a little carried away here, but the point is that, depending on the number of patients sharing similar clinical and nonclinical characteristics, fairly specific populations can be created, and by doing so, even greater quality and cost-efficiency outcomes can be achieved.

The definition of a PHM population, therefore, is often multi-factorial rather than based on a single patient characteristic, allowing for even greater value realization. Only through the bookends of individualization of patients (that is, Aim #3) and population health (Aim #2) can we realize true, high value health and healthcare.

Aim #3 is unique in another way relative to its two precedents: it specifically calls for *cost reduction.* The other two Aims (Improve the Patient Experience of Care and Improve the Health of Populations) are more vague and are concerned with the numerator in the value equation, *quality.* Aim #3 is both very specific and a not-so-subtle reminder that reducing the equation's denominator—the *cost* of healthcare—is critical, lest we fail to truly achieve meaningful, sustainable healthcare reform. *Aim #3 is a check on the two preceding Aims,* reminding us that while we must improve the health of our populations and we must improve the patient experience, these goals must be achieved only in cost-efficient ways. *Bookends.*

Aim #3 is a check on the two preceding Aims, reminding us that while we must improve the health of our populations and we must improve the patient experience, these goals must be achieved only in cost-efficient ways.

 PEARL

Aim #3 emphasizes that we appreciate a patient's *individual* medical and nonmedical characteristics and challenges. This Aim also demands we recognize the importance of cost efficiency in pursuing the two previous Aims.

Finally, as we have for the previous two Aims, we must for this final Aim answer the question of *"Who?"* Individualizing patients (whether for the stated goal of cost reduction or to better create populations) requires significant physician input because understanding medical conditions and the interrelationships between medical comorbidities is a physician specialty. However, as with the previous two Aims, *nurses and allied health professionals must play a major role* in individualization by virtue of their unique, deep, broad connections with their patients and families. Nurses and allied health professionals frequently get to know their patients more deeply as individual people. Understanding and appreciating patients *individually* on such a personal, socio-economic-demographic level empowers these providers in the critical process of *population health* management.

Nurses, Allied Health Professionals, and the Triple Aim: In Summary

Our destination is far ahead, over the horizon. Consistent, sustainable, high-quality, cost-efficient, out-of-hospital preventive and maintenance healthcare. Whether or not we think it is the best GPS system, our current roadmap is The Triple Aim. Thus, we are directed to consider the *experience* of those for whom we are privileged to care not only in terms of the clinical care we provide, but also more globally in overall care, communications, and compassion. We are no longer to focus on the physician (the true focus of the traditional "doctor-patient relationship"); rather we must center all care delivery around our patients, both as individuals and as members of one or more patient populations. We are to consider both value (which includes clinical quality and patient experience) and cost.

Our healthcare reform GPS is The Triple Aim, and nurses and allied health professionals will need to do much of the driving if we are to reach our destination.

● **PEARL**

Nurses and allied health professionals will play a major role in achieving all three Aims.

References

1. Institute for Healthcare Improvement (online) 2017; http://www.ihi.org/engage/initiatives/TripleAim/Pages/default.aspx.
2. Barr P. *Patient Experience Is Increasingly Important*. Hospitals & Health Networks (online); 2016. http://www.hhnmag.com/articles/7083-patient-experience-is-increasingly-important.

3. Rene Letourneau. *Better HCAHPS Scores Protect Revenue*. HealthLeaders Media (online); 2016. http://www.healthleadersmedia.com/finance/better-hcahps-scores-protect-revenue.
4. HCAHPS (online); http://www.hcahpsonline.org/home.aspx.
5. Centers for Medicare and Medicaid Services (online); https://www.cms.gov/medicare/quality-initiatives-patient-assessment-instruments/hospitalqualityinits/hospitalhcahps.html.
6. Medicare.gov (onine); https://www.medicare.gov/hospitalcompare/Data/Overview.html.
7. Centers for Medicare and Medicaid Services (online); https://www.cms.gov/Research-Statistics-Data-and-Systems/Research/CAHPS/OAS-CAHPS.html.
8. Rodak S. *Should Hospitals Treat Patients as Customers, Partners or Both?* Becker's Hospital Review (online); 2012. http://www.beckershospitalreview.com/strategic-planning/should-hospitals-treat-patients-as-customers-partners-or-both.html.
9. Hixon T. *Are we Patients, Consumers, or Customers?* Forbes (online); 2015. https://www.forbes.com/sites/toddhixon/2015/10/22/are-we-patients-consumers-or-customers/#3f840be01434.
10. HCAHPSonline.org (online); http://www.hcahpsonline.org/files/HCAHPS%20V9.0%20Appendix%20A%20-%20Mail%20Survey%20Materials%20(English)%20March%202014.pdf.
11. Aiken LH, Sermeus W, Van den Heede K, et al. Patient safety, satisfaction, and quality of hospital care: cross sectional surveys of nurses and patients in 12 Countries in Europe and the United States. *Br Med J.* 2012;344. e1717.
12. Chan KY, Wang W, Wu JJ, et al. Epidemiology of Alzheimer's disease and other forms of dementia in China, 1990–2010: a systematic review and analysis. *Lancet.* 2013;381:201–2023.
13. Keogh-Brown MR, Jensen HT, et al. The growing macroeconomic burden of Alzheimer's Disease in China. *Alzheimer's Dementia.* 2015;11:1810182.
14. National Cancer Institute of Brazil (INCA) (online; in Portuguese) 2015; http://www2.inca.gov.br/wps/wcm/connect/acoes_programas/site/home/nobrasil/programa_nacional_controle_cancer_colo_utero/conceito_magnitude.
15. Dictionary.com (online); http://www.dictionary.com/browse/per-capita?s=t.
16. Cardiovascular Disease and Diabetes. American Heart Association (online) 2016; http://www.heart.org/HEARTORG/Conditions/More/Diabetes/WhyDiabetesMatters/Cardiovascular-Disease-Diabetes_UCM_313865_Article.jsp/#.WMKwH_Kkz30.

CHAPTER **6**

Patient Engagement: The New Frontier

Up to now, we've spent a great deal of time talking about *healthcare.* As I said in Chapter 2, in the airline analogy of our traditional care delivery model, the patient is often little more than the passive airplane passenger. Patients and their loved ones often play only minor roles in the healthcare decisions that directly impact their health and their lives (if they play any role at all). But the problem with the passive patient model goes deeper than just an absence of decision-making input. *Far deeper.* And if we don't correct this problem, if we don't radically alter our society's perception of the role of the patient, there simply is no way that we'll ever achieve truly meaningful healthcare reform, because the biggest reason that the value of our healthcare system is so poor (both quality and cost-efficiency) is not our *healthcare.* It's our *health.*

And the individuals most responsible of our population's terrible health are not our physicians or our nurses or our allied health professionals or our health system administrators or even our politicians. *We are the people most responsible for our terrible health.* We Americans. *We are why our health is so lousy.*

The biggest reason that the quality of our healthcare system is so poor and the biggest reason that our healthcare spending is out of control is not our *healthcare*. It is our *health*. And *we are the people most responsible for our terrible health.*

Now I understand that this is a generalization, but all you need to do is take a walk down the street, sit in a movie theater, go to a mall, and for many of us, simply look at our own diet and behaviors, and it will be obvious: as a society, we do not take very good care of our bodies or our health.

It's a very strange thing, really. Our American culture expects and even demands that we all take responsibility as individuals and accept accountability for every major decision and action that we take in living our lives. *Except when it comes to our own health.* Every homeowner is responsible and accountable for selecting and then paying his or her mortgage. Same for everyone who rents their residence. Every individual with a job is responsible for showing up for work on time and performing the duties in their job description. Mothers and fathers are accountable for raising and providing for their children and ensuring that those children behave appropriately. Our car payments. Buying our food. Paying our bills. Following the laws. We individuals are responsible and accountable for all of our decisions or actions, and we face consequences for failing to meet those obligations (and benefits for fulfilling those requirements). Yet when it comes to decisions, behaviors, and activities that have an impact our own individual health, *we as individuals and a society completely and utterly fail to "own our health."* Obese? Oh, well! Diabetes resulting from obesity? So be it! COPD from smoking? It is what it is! Repeated hospitalizations for uncontrolled heart failure? Nothing I could do!

> When it comes to decisions, behaviors, and activities that impact our own individual health, *we as individuals and a society completely and utterly fail to "own our health."*

It is extremely unlikely that you would offer to chip in to help pay the cost of rebuilding your neighbor's house knowing that he accidentally burned it to the ground in a drunken stupor. But you are expected to pay for his failing liver when his alcoholism leads to cirrhosis. Or for the dialysis required to keep a diabetic alive, even though that diabetes is entirely the result of obesity, a poor diet, and

PEARL

The biggest driver of our low quality, high cost healthcare is *the poor health of our population.*

failure to get off the couch. When it comes to health, we are "our brother's keeper;" that is, we are expected to pay for care resulting from the poor health choices and behaviors of others.[1] Note that I am *not* talking about the "social determinants" of health,[2] such as an individual's financial, educational, and housing status, which *are not* under the direct control of that individual. I am speaking of "choices and behaviors" that clearly *are* under the direct control of the individual. But is it that simple? More and more the evidence suggests that it is not, that there are links between some social determinants and individual behavioral choices that have long been viewed as unrelated.[3,4]

That said, whether or not some behavioral choices are interdependent with social determinants, *until our entire society undergoes a paradigm shift and accepts the responsibility and accountability of the individual patient as the primary owner of his or her health choices and behaviors* (that is, recognizing the *Patient as Provider*), we will never fully realize meaningful improvement in our population's health.

> Until our entire society undergoes a paradigm shift and accepts the responsibility and accountability of the individual as the primary owner of his or her health choices and behaviors, we will never fully realize meaningful improvement in our population's health.

Our unwillingness to hold ourselves and each other responsible and accountable, to demand that individuals own their health as we own our mortgages and our family responsibilities, combined with our failure to as a society adequately drive improvement in social determinants linked to unhealthy behavioral choices, results in two dramatic, negative consequences. First, our health as a population continues to deteriorate, leading to an unnecessarily poor quality of life and shorter lifespans[5-7] for far too many Americans (consider the obesity epidemic alone). Second, as is the case with preventable medical errors at the hands of providers, our preventable health crisis costs us (the public) ever increasing truckloads of money as we pay to diagnose and (attempt to) treat all of these avoidable conditions (including the significant indirect costs, such as loss of work productivity). And the total cost of poor behavioral decisions (such as smoking, poor diet, no exercise) is also *enormous,* totaling in the *high hundreds of billions of dollars each and every year.*[8-10]

If we are honest with ourselves, many of us as individuals, and America as a population, as a society, we all are far-and-away the most responsible for our current health and healthcare disaster. By refusing to "Own Our Health" as we own our mortgages, work responsibilities, and child rearing, we have directly reduced the quality of our health and accelerated the cost of our healthcare.

Of Cars and Healthcare

> **PEARL**
>
> Our unhealthy nation is in a large part the result of patients (at some point, *each and every one of us*) failing to truly own their health (accept responsibility and accountability for their health-related decisions and behaviors).

In virtually every state in the United States, it is illegal to operate a car unless the driver and all passengers (at least front seat) have fastened their seat belts.[11] And yet every year, tens of thousands of fathers, mothers, daughters, and sons are killed, and hundreds of thousands are injured, all because they fail to buckle up. According to the Centers for Disease Control and Prevention, of the more than 32,000 US drivers and passengers killed in auto accidents, "about half" had failed to buckle their seat belts.[12] Everyone knows: *seat belts save lives.* And yet hundreds of thousands of drivers and passengers voluntarily ignore the well-known risks and fail to perform this simple, 2-second task, suffering (along with their loved ones) the tragic consequences.

No, you haven't accidentally picked up *Death on the Highway* off of the coffee table. But this real-world seat belt analogy is helpful in understanding not only the failure of our traditional healthcare system, but a major risk to successful healthcare reform. *Simply mandating high quality healthcare* as the Affordable Care Act (ACA or "ObamaCare") does, just as simply mandating seat belt use, fails to automatically translate into better quality care for patients (or safety for all drivers and passengers). But where the ACA *really* fails is in how far the healthcare law actually deviates from our seat belt analogy; that is, in *the target of the legislation.* While seat belt laws specifically target those who directly benefit from the safety legislation (drivers and passengers), *healthcare insurance reform legislation does not target those who are both largely in control of their health and the beneficiaries of better quality healthcare: patients.* (It can be argued that the ACA's "Individual Mandate" is a nudge towards patient compliance by taxing individuals who fail to purchase basic health insurance; however, the law only allows the tax to be *voluntarily paid* or withheld from an Internal Revenue Service tax refund. The uninsured individual is *not open to prosecution, liens, or levies.*)[13]

Now consider these two statistics:

1. On average, an American visits his or her doctor four times a year[14]
2. On average, an American physician spends 13 to 16 minutes interacting with the patient per visit[15] (and *more than 37% of an ambulatory patient interaction is spent with the physician is focused on the electronic health record (EHR)* and other documentation activities, *not on the patient*)[16]

Let's do the simple math (using the generous 16-minute statistic):

$$4 \times 16 = 64$$

In other words, *on average, Americans spend only about 64 minutes a year in the presence of a physician* (and again, much of that time, the physician is not focused on the patient). Yep, just over an hour. (Imagine the favorable impact on our health if we spent only 64 minutes a year at fast food restaurants or only 64 minutes a year with our butts planted on the couch in front of the television.) Now, of course, there are many folks who spend time in the hospital, where they interact much more frequently and for a much greater total duration with providers, but in many cases, the need for hospitalization represents at least in part a failure of the patient to prevent or control their condition (medication noncompliance, etc.). At the other end of the spectrum are the millions of Americans who see a doctor less than four times annually (often *far less often*).

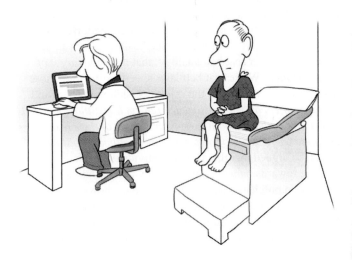

So from a realistic time perspective, physicians and nurses and health providers can have little (to no) meaningful impact on the health of our population as a whole. Your medical assistant can't come to your house twice a day to force you to take your blood pressure pill. Your nurse can't chase you into your bathroom and demand that you get onto the bathroom scale. Your dietician can't follow you around, snatching the donut and chips out of your hand. The simple truth here, folks, is that *virtually all of the routine decisions, behaviors, and actions that have an impact on an individual's health (both favorably and unfavorably) are enacted far from the influence of any healthcare provider:* when we're at work, out to dinner, watching a movie, listening to our child's band concert . . .

On average, Americans spend only about 64 minutes a year in the presence of a physician. Imagine the favorable impact on our health if we spent only 64 minutes a year at fast food restaurants or only 64 minutes a year with our butts planted on the couch in front of the television.

But does this matter to any of us? I mean, if my neighbor fails to get screened and ends up having surgery, then radiation therapy, and then chemotherapy for his colon cancer, isn't that *his problem?* Yes, from a quality (and even quantity) of life perspective, his poor decision hurts only him (and those who care about him). But from a *cost perspective,* his individual decision to hurt the quality of his own individual life *hurts us all.* Our entire population. Our society. The refusal by individuals to accept accountability and responsibility for their own health is *emptying all of our wallets and our bank accounts.* For those patients without insurance or adequate insurance, the cost to us all is direct. But much of the cost to society is indirect, for example: elevated taxes, increased insurance premiums, and lost work productivity. This last one, lost work productivity, is a biggie.[17] Businesses lose over $560 *billion* every year when people are too ill to work and in Workers Compensation payments.[18] Again, let's harken back to our previous shoplifting analogy. *Businesses pass those costs on to the consumer.* To you and me. So through both direct and indirect routes, your neighbor's failure to take care of his or her health results in *your paying more* of your hard-earned money. Who do you think pays for that smoker's lung cancer operation? *You and I do.* Who do you think pays for that obesity-induced diabetic's dialysis? *You and I do.* Who do you think pays for that flu victim's hospitalization, that patient who chose to forgo a flu shot? *You and I do.* Through state and federal taxes and through our own insurance premiums, you and I pay for the healthcare needs of those unable to pay for their own healthcare.[19]

> From a cost perspective, an individual's decision to hurt the quality of his or her own individual life *hurts us all.*

And yet the ACA overwhelmingly (many would argue *entirely,* given the economic inefficiency of the Individual Mandate[20]) aims its penalties *not at patients, but at healthcare providers:* hospitals and healthcare delivery systems and their clinical staff.[21-23] In doing so, in failing to demand that patients "buckle up," *the current reform legislation fails to provide a powerful incentive to those in the strongest position to dramatically and sustainably increase the value of health on a national scale.* Thus, while it is likely that today's approach of financially penalizing healthcare providers (often severely) for failing to deliver government-defined, value-based care may somewhat improve care quality and costs, *unless patients themselves accept ownership of their own personal health and healthcare, our society as a whole has no realistic shot at dramatically improving our current, untenable, unhealthy healthcare system.*

> Unless patients themselves accept ownership of their own personal health and healthcare, our society as a whole has no realistic shot at dramatically improving our current, untenable, unhealthy healthcare system.

The Riddle

As individuals, we own our financial responsibilities (our loans, mortgages, taxes). We own our employment responsibilities (showing up to work on time, doing our job). We own our family responsibilities (caring for the safety, health, education, and nurturing of our children). We own every single major aspect of our adult lives.

Except for our health.

An enormous portion of our population fails to "own their health." As with the father who doesn't ensure that his children are buckled up before racing down the highway, *it's an intellectually perplexing riddle:* why is there such an enormous disconnect between the obese, diabetic woman still sucking down Big Gulps and the heart attack, leg amputation, and dialysis she has been told are likely waiting down the line? Or that chain-smoking man with advanced COPD and a chronic cough who wouldn't think of failing to pay his monthly cell phone bill yet shrugs off any suggestion that he consider a smoking reduction program?

But this riddle is more complex than just asking why individuals refuse to accept responsibility for their own health. We're all part of the riddle. Therapists, nurses, physicians, even insurers . . . *seemingly everyone* accepts as *fait accompli* the damaged quality of life and financial waste that results from our own individual voluntary behavioral and clinical choices. And it is this riddle, *our society's refusal to expect individuals to own their health,* which poses *the single greatest obstacle to true, sustainable, widespread improvement in our nation's health and healthcare.*

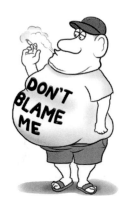

It is this riddle, our society's refusal to expect individuals to own their health, which poses the single greatest obstacle to true, sustainable, widespread improvement in our nation's health and healthcare.

Surely our government—faced with the disastrous economic implications of a greater than 17% gross domestic product (GDP) healthcare spending that continues to rocket skyward—will step in! After all, the new healthcare laws already financially punish those providers who fail to meet ACA care standards.[21-23] So *why don't our politicians aggressively penalize the millions of patients who refuse to even moderately alter their health-damaging decisions and behaviors?* Why doesn't our government heavily tax that obese diabetic who fails to improve her diet or at least regularly check her blood sugar level? Why isn't there a law punishing that smoker for refusing to at least attempt a smoking reduction program?

The cynical answer? Because these people, and tens of millions more just like them, are *voters.*

And there is support for this cynical view. Search the internet and learn what happened when the governor of the Great State of Texas signed an executive order mandating childhood vaccination against human papilloma virus (HPV) to protect girls from future cervical cancers and genital warts . . . (If you're too busy to Google this, I'll tell you: enough voters rebelled against the governor's mandate that the state legislature overturned the executive order.[24] Many other states have, like Texas, abandoned initial attempts at requiring HPV vaccination, while other states with less conservative populations have enacted such legislation.)[25]

Still, this cynical answer only suggests why *politicians* might be unwilling to hold individuals accountable for voluntary actions (or inactions) that elevate everyone's costs. What about *patients themselves?* What about *physicians, nurses,* and *allied health professionals? Why do we all simply accept that patients aren't accountable or responsible for their own health* (and associated healthcare costs)?

Such a dissection of the depths of the American psyche— while critical to achieve and sustain high value healthcare— is far outside of the scope of this tome. In other words: I'm sorry, this book will not solve this master riddle.

Still, there *is* something we can do that will help drive health ownership. We can focus not on the *Why* (the focus of the riddle), but on the *How* and the *Who.* That is, *How do we drive health ownership* (individual acceptance of accountability and responsibility for one's own health and healthcare), and *Who will drive* the health ownership movement?

Patient Engagement: The Complexity Behind the Buzzword

"Healthcare Reform." "Population Health." "Value-Based Reimbursement." "Patient Engagement."

These are all powerful, action-oriented terms that sit at the heart of today's drive towards better health. But the danger inherent in these and other such "buzzwords" is that they hide the enormous challenges, tremendous complexity, and voluminous details inherent within the processes they label.

"Patient Engagement" is a fundamental principle of health ownership. Only when enough individual Americans demonstrate active interest and involvement in the decisions, behaviors, and activities that have a direct impact on their own health and healthcare (i.e., when they become *health owners*) will we move the larger healthcare reform needle in the right direction. Yet even simply agreeing on a definition of "Patient Engagement" has proven difficult. But that said, let's dive into Patient Engagement, which if clearly defined (whether or not that definition is uniformly accepted), properly understood, and even partially successfully implemented, offers an enormous opportunity to improve the health of our population.

● PEARL

Only through successful, broad, and deep *Patient Engagement, Patient Education,* and *Patient Empowerment* can we have an impact on the value of our healthcare in a meaningful way.

But you might ask, "Why is Patient Engagement so critical a topic for allied health professionals and nurses? That is, why are we discussing it in such detail in this book?"

It is precisely *because* it is so critical to improved population health and to meaningful healthcare reform that *nurses and allied health professionals must be the primary drivers of Patient Engagement.*

The Three Phases of "Patient Engagement"

"Patient Engagement" itself is both the highest level umbrella term and the first of *three sequential phases* underneath that umbrella that describe the journey towards health ownership. The complete journey moves from *Patient Engagement* to *Patient Education* to *Patient Empowerment.*

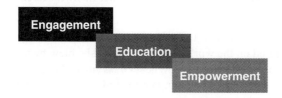

Several important points here. First, to reiterate, *these three phases must be sequential.* There can be no truly successful Patient Education *unless patients are first engaged;* that is, patients must be truly interested in better understanding their own health and healthcare. Nor can patients and their loved ones truly be empowered to own their health *if they are not first educated* about their own specific behavioral options, clinical conditions, and clinical choices.

Second, in our wonderfully entrepreneurial world, we already have available numerous useful and powerful Patient Education and Patient Empowerment solutions (and more continue to enter the commercial market).

And third, *many people confuse "Patient Education" and "Patient Empowerment" with "Patient Engagement."* This is a significant mistake (which we'll discuss further in a moment), for not only is meaningful "Patient Engagement" *the trigger* for this three-phase cascade, but it is far-and-away *the most difficult aspect of health ownership* and, therefore, the key to patient-driven sustainable healthcare reform.

 PEARL

The three phases of "Patient Engagement" are *sequential.* Powerful Patient Education and Patient Empowerment solutions are already widely available.

Patient Education: A (Quick) Overview

We are fortunate that today's healthcare technology sector already offers a trove of Patient Education solutions. And while nurses and allied health professionals certainly must participate in guiding patient utilization of these educational tools, the critical role of providers in Patient *Engagement* deserves far more of our attention here. Still, let's start with a quick look at the second phase of health ownership.

> Theresa sat in front of her laptop, her eyes burning holes into the screen. A self-described "Type A" personality, she had immediately planted herself in front of her computer the moment she returned home from her doctor's office. The needle biopsy had confirmed her doctor's suspicion: Theresa had thyroid cancer. Not one to sit still, let alone wallow in fear or self-pity, she hadn't even bothered to take off her coat before initiating her internet search for "thyroid cancer."

> Theresa was smart. She knew there was a lot of crap offered on the worldwide web. Thus, she blew by the website claiming that "Wheat Grass Juice Cures Thyroid Cancer!" instead clicking on the link to a world-renowned medical center.

> There it was. Page after page in plain English, and dozens of images, all explaining the incidence, symptoms, diagnosis, work-up, treatment options, follow-up, and prognosis for patients with the very same malignancy that she harbored in her neck.

> Theresa took in a deep breath before slowly exhaling. *She was fully engaged and ready to be educated.* She clicked on "Thyroid Cancer: An Overview."

> Within seconds, her shoulders sagged, and she let out an audible sigh. There on the page before her were descriptions of *four types of thyroid cancer.* A rapid perusal confirmed her fear: there were meaningful differences in the behavior, treatment, and prognosis of the differing types.

> Did she have *papillary* thyroid cancer? *Follicular? Medullary?* Or (God forbid) *anaplastic?* She didn't know . . . Maybe her physician had told her, but as soon as he had said "cancer," Theresa's mind had raced ahead, his words a muffled background.

She clicked onto the "Evaluation" page.

Even worse . . .

Even assuming that she had the most common type (papillary), *there were six different cancer stages,* each with its own treatment options and prognosis. She had no idea what stage she had . . .

This simple but all-too-common example reminds us of several critical points. If Theresa wasn't engaged in her own health and healthcare, she wouldn't even have browsed the internet. *A patient must first be engaged to be educated* (much more on this in a moment.) But *even the fully engaged patient initially needs to be educated with some basic information specific to their own individual clinical situation.* If Theresa's physician had written down the information (or if she had brought a friend with her who could have served as a scribe), she would have known her cancer type and stage (or the plan for staging her disease), an initial education that would have allowed this engaged patient to independently further educate herself on her own. This would then have prepared Theresa to move into the Patient Empowerment phase, providing her a sense of control over her own care management decisions; that is, *true health ownership* that empowers a meaningful patient-provider partnership (creating a positive "patient experience") resulting in higher quality, more cost-efficient healthcare.

> Even the fully engaged patient initially needs to be educated with some basic information specific to his or her own individual clinical situation.

Unfortunately, whether due to overly busy providers and/or to the failure of patients to seek clarity when they don't clearly understand the provided information, patients (even if engaged) are all too often lacking in the basic education specific to their scenario that is required to empower autonomous further learning. Sometimes there are opportunities for nurses and allied health professionals to provide the necessary patient-specific knowledge or confirm that the information is clearly understood, allowing the engaged patient to enter the Education phase. But often such information is not within the non-physician provider's area of expertise. In such cases, the nurse or allied health professional can truly help the patient by respectfully reminding the physician of the need to confirm that the patient possesses and understands the appropriate initial, basic information concerning his or her clinical situation.

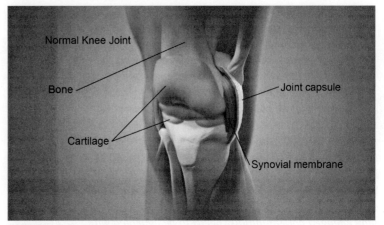

FIGURE 6.1 Targeted patient education solutions come in a variety of languages, educational levels, and presentation formats.

Today's Patient Education solutions are *amazing.* The post-myocardial infarction, type 2 diabetic can learn in his or her own primary *language,* at his or her own *educational level,* and in his or her own preferred delivery *format* (text, image, video) about preventive and health maintenance activities *specific to his or her medical condition and comorbidities.* Rapid, easy-to-use educational solutions are available across the internet (although website credibility is a significant issue); even better, current, credible, evidence-based information is often offered for free by many provider facilities and health systems (Fig. 6.1).

But again, don't confuse targeted, individualized, language/educational/format-specific Patient *Education* with Patient *Engagement.* If they are unused or minimally used, not understood or poorly understood, such potentially powerful patient educational solutions are simply *the clinical equivalent of unbuckled seatbelts,* providing little or no opportunity for risk and cost-of-care reduction if the patient doesn't first buckle up (first *engage*).

Engage first, *then* educate.

Patient Empowerment: A (Quicker) Overview

"Mom," I pleaded with my 83-year-old mother, "Can we please get going? I have to pick up the girls."

"Just give me one moment," she said, her head still bent downward, her eyes holding their focus on her smartphone screen. "I just need to text your aunt and then deposit some checks into my savings account."

I rolled my eyes and sighed (she didn't notice, or pretended not to).

Forty seconds later, she looked up and smiled. "All done!"

Listen, when my octogenarian mother (who still doesn't trust microwave ovens or ATMs) can use her cell phone or laptop to ask a question of her physical therapist or infusion nurse, look up images to match with any one of her dozen-or-so prescription medications, compare quality outcomes of two nearby hospitals, and schedule a visit to get her flu shot, then we truly are already in *The Age of Patient Empowerment.* Our tech-savvy population is fully capable of adopting and utilizing the hundreds of available Patient Empowerment tools; that is, simple, intuitive, mobile technology that delivers targeted Patient Education, allows for real-time communication with providers, and facilitates numerous other health and healthcare empowerment activities (Fig. 6.2).

And now, let's get to the heart (and challenge) of health ownership . . .

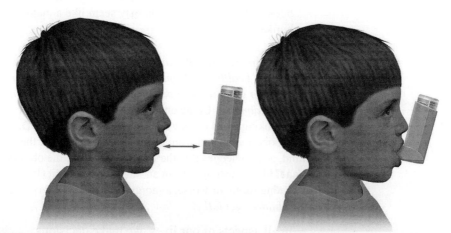

FIGURE 6.2 Patient empowerment solutions allow for the delivery of patient education, for communication with providers, and for engagement in other health ownership opportunities.

Successful Patient Engagement: The How and the Who

Forget about healthcare for a moment. Forget that you're a nurse or a physical therapist or a pharmacy technician or whatever serves as your professional identity. Think of yourself simply as *a person.*

How do you, how do each of us, make decisions?

Whether we consciously realize it or not, in virtually every aspect of our lives, we make decisions large and small by *balancing the potential benefits against the potential risks or burdens.*

> You and your spouse just love that 3500-square foot, two-story colonial at the end of the cul-de-sac. What's not to love?! It's a beautiful home! It's a fantastic location! But . . . can you afford the monthly mortgage payments? In a nutshell, *do the benefits* the house offers *outweigh the financial burdens* of buying it?

> Yikes! You're running late for work, and this morning is a rarity: the boss herself is leading the first-thing-in-the-morning meeting! *Is the benefit* of being bright-eyed and bushy-tailed when your boss first enters the meeting room *worth the risk* of a speeding ticket or, worse yet, an accident?

> How about this one? *Right now* you could be at the movies, out to dinner, enjoying a hike, taking a nap . . . . truly positive activities. Instead, you're reading this book, which to some of you may seem like a major burden . . .

My point here is that *only when it relates to our own health and healthcare do many of us completely abandon our risk-benefit scale when choosing how we behave and what we do or don't do.* Come on: every smoker clearly knows that smoking leads to lung cancer, heart disease, COPD. Every obese man and woman, at least in the back of their mind, acknowledges that the light at the end of the obesity tunnel likely is shining from an intensive care unit (ICU), operating room, or worse, a morgue. And still, *we even let our children get fat!*

> In all aspects of our lives, we make decisions large and small by balancing the potential benefits against the potential risks or burdens.

As noted previously, this *riddle*—this disconnect—between the perceived benefits of our choices and the known likely or potential negative health consequences of those choices is mind-boggling. It's like an out-of-body experience shared by the majority of our population (and much of the human race). And while we don't necessarily have to understand the *Why* of this riddle, we must be able to solve the *How* if we as a society are ever to achieve consistent, sustainable, high-value health and healthcare, and the best way to solve the *How* of the riddle is through meaningful, widespread Patient Engagement.

So, *how are we to engage* the man with hypertension who has no symptoms, and for whom the prescribed medication causes impotence and general fatigue? Is he simply to accept his provider's word, that although entirely asymptomatic, he is actually suffering from a dangerous condition that *potentially* could lead to a heart attack or stroke? To the man with no symptoms, these are only *potential risks.* And potential risks *in the future.* But *the burdens* of the immediate, recommended medical treatment and behavioral modifications *are neither potential nor futuristic.* They are *real,* and they are *now*, and they are forever. He now must remember to take his medication daily (a minimal burden, but a burden nonetheless). A medication that renders him impotent (a major burden for most men). A medication that makes him constantly feel tired (another major burden). And he has been instructed to give up some of the food that he has loved to eat his entire life (another major burden). And he is supposed to start walking several times a week (also a burden for this couch potato). All because *maybe, someday, there's a chance* that he could suffer a heart attack or a stroke.

But *there is help,* we providers assure ourselves. We'll simply provide this man with the powerful American Heart Association/American Stroke Association *High Blood Pressure Health Risk Calculator* (Figure 6.3) internet URL,[26] allowing our patient and his wife to become *educated* and *empowered* in reducing his risk of heart attack, stroke, heart failure, and kidney disease. *In just minutes! For free!*

This and similar powerful educational and empowerment tools (combined in this tool) are easy to find, simple to use, and (when from credible sources) reliable in guiding patients to healthier lives. But anyone who cares for patients knows that for the many (perhaps the majority) of patients, *simply providing the URL and a few words of encouragement will likely never result in that patient going to the site, let alone using the Risk Calculator.* Let alone *altering his or*

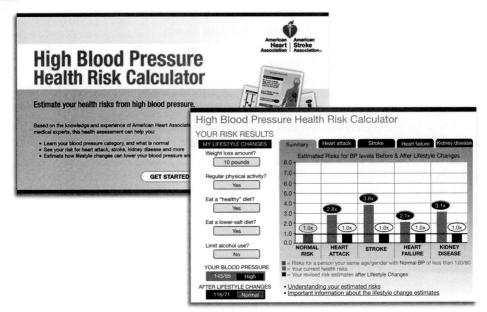

FIGURE 6.3 The AHA/ASA High Blood Pressure Health Risk Calculator allows a patient in only a few minutes to learn about risks specific to him or her and to appreciate the real reduction in those risks that can result from specific, voluntary clinical, and behavioral. (From High Blood Pressure Health Risk Calculator. American Heart Association/American Stroke Association [online]; http://tools.bigbeelabs.com/aha/tools/hbp/.)

her lifestyle to reduce the risk of heart attack, stroke, heart failure, and kidney disease. Because providing guidance to an internet site (or journal, book, magazine) *does not guarantee engagement.* And without engagement, patient education and empowerment cannot be realized in any meaningful way.

Thus, we still have failed to answer the *How* question. How to engage the patient so that the patient then becomes engaged and, ultimately, educated and empowered. But the answer to the *How* question is intimately linked to the *Who* question.

And two of the main answers to the *Who* question are: *nurses* and *allied health professionals.*

Why not physicians?

"Hi, Mr. Parsons. I'm Dr. Edelstein, your surgeon. I'd like to spend the next 90 minutes speaking with you and your wife about your asymptomatic high blood pressure. I'm certain that as we get to truly know one another, together we will be able to share a journey to a healthier future through changes in your diet and activities, and with the addition of some medications. So, let's start out by you sharing with me . . ."

Come on, people. Not only don't most physicians function in this manner, the healthcare system is most efficient when each provider "works at the top of his or her license." This means that providers should overwhelmingly engage in activities that represent the most advanced, skilled activities that they can provide. Surgeons bring far greater value to patients (and payers) when in the operating room rather than when spending long periods of time speaking with patients and families (activities that not only can be performed, but are *frequently performed better,* by non-physicians).[27] Now, don't get me wrong. We should all (physicians included) demonstrate a true interest in our patients and their loved ones as people and as individuals. We should all (physicians included) spend time interacting with our patients, getting to know them on a personal level. But when it comes to the allocation of limited, highly skilled resources, physicians in general most benefit patients and payers through the direct provision of medical and/or surgical care.

Now go back and read that little clinical scenario about Mr. Parsons, above. Go ahead . . . I'll wait.

In actuality, the interest that this fictional physician demonstrates in Mr. Parsons and his family is *exactly what a provider needs to do to engage patients:* get to know the patient as an individual person.

The Solution to the Patient Engagement Riddle

Many patients (perhaps most) can indeed become truly engaged in their own health, allowing them to then proceed through education and on to empowerment. The results can be dramatic not only for the individual, but for our entire population (once enough individuals are engaged, educated, and empowered). Below, I lay out the basic steps that a provider (you!) can take to initiate and drive successful patient engagement. Recognize that to successfully encourage a person to own his or her health is not a tightly scripted process. You must use your own style and interpersonal skills to connect with the patient and advance the engagement process. In some cases, engagement may occur quickly, while at other times, the seeds of engagement may only begin to germinate after several conversations. And in other instances, patients simply will not engage despite your best efforts (more on this later in this chapter).

The Basic Steps for a Provider to Initiate Meaningful Patient Engagement

1. *Get to know the individual as a person, not as a patient, condition, or disease.*

2. *Include and engage the patient's loved ones, friends, clergy, or whoever can help in supporting improved health and healthcare* for the patient. Remember, they spend far more time with the patient than you ever will, and they have a deeper investment in the patient remaining healthy than you do.

3. *Begin with the nonclinical, nonmedical conversations.* Learn about the person's life, particularly *what they enjoy* (golfing every Saturday, visiting National Parks, movies) and *what they are planning and hoping to do in the future* (traveling after retirement, a child's wedding, a grandchild's graduation).

4. Then when you feel the time is right, begin to *positively link behavioral choices that the individual can make* (with the strong support of loved ones) *with benefits relating to what you have learned that individual values* currently (golf, movies) and for the future (travel, family events, grandchildren).

5. *Together, utilize technological solutions* (including credible websites) to further engage the patient and loved ones in owning his or her health and healthcare. *A balance of personal involvement (you) and technology can be very powerful* in engaging patients.

6. *Speak in positive rather than in negative terms.* "You'll really help your heart and your health by making this change in your diet" is more motivating than "You'll risk dying of a heart attack if you don't change your diet."

7. Don't go for the big sell! Behavioral changes (such as weight loss, improving the diet, getting off the couch and taking a walk, medication compliance) are difficult. Thus encourage behavioral changes in an *appropriately paced, iterative, and incremental fashion.* For example, go from rarely walking to walking down the driveway twice a week, then later to three times a week, then later to a slightly longer walk down the street twice weekly, and so on. Base the pace of advancement on what you've learned of the person and by encouraging that person and his or her loved ones to help create a realistic but forward-moving plan.

8. Finally, Patient Engagement routinely requires repeated provider involvement and encouragement; that is, for most patients, engagement isn't a "one and done" deal.

Rather, on every provider visit, try to carve out time to review and reinforce the positive benefits of the patient's health ownership activities.

Back to our previous example, using the numbered steps from above:

#1 and #2. In *taking the time* to speak with your asymptomatic hypertensive patient and his wife and in *demonstrating warmth and sincere personal interest in them,* you've made a connection.

#3. You've learned that the couple is already planning their first trip to Europe after the patient's planned retirement in 2 years. Their eldest daughter is expecting her first child in 4 months, and their younger daughter is now in her freshman year at Stanford.

#4. Sensing that the time is right, you begin to explain how, with truly achievable, iterative, and incremental behavioral choices—and with the strong support of his wife—your patient can better ensure that he'll be healthy when his grandchild is born, his daughter graduates, and when the time arrives to take that postretirement trip to Europe.

#5, #6, and #7. *Together,* the three of you create a realistic (for him) approach to reducing his risk of heart attack and stroke by *together* working through the American Heart Association/American Stroke Association *High Blood Pressure Health Risk Calculator. Together,* you work through the *Risk Calculator*, making appropriately conservative choices regarding positive dietary and exercise changes. *Together,* you celebrate the clear, favorable impact the *Calculator* states that those changes will have on reducing his heart attack and stroke risks, again linking these risk reductions to the couple's positive, personal plans.

Then you have an open, honest discussion about his medication. You acknowledge that the side effects he is experiencing are a real problem. You encourage your patient and his wife to speak in the same open, honest fashion with his physician, with the goal of identifying a medication with a better side effect profile (and explaining that he may need to try a few antihypertensive agents to find the drug that is best for him).

Finally, you again move away from the clinical and just talk. You make it clear that you look forward to hearing about the new baby, the graduation, the travel. And you share that you are available to talk about his health and healthcare choices whenever he or his wife wish.

#8. When you next see the patient and his wife in the office 3 months later, you are pleased to hear how his children are doing, how their plans for postretirement are coming along, and how he is feeling. You discuss his new medication and review his progress with the dietary and exercise plan you previously created together. You discuss areas where he is succeeding and areas where he feels challenged, modifying the plan as seems appropriate. And you congratulate him and his wife on their success so far, reminding him of the personal benefits that he, his wife, and his entire family are achieving through his own involvement in his health.

Two takeaways that are worth reemphasizing:

1. Patient Engagement demands that a provider *takes adequate time* to engage the patient (and more often than not, the patient's loved ones)
2. Patient Engagement requires that a provider *demonstrates sincere interest* in getting to know the patient *as a person.*

For many patients, it is *when a provider personally, compassionately links the individual's own health choices with that individual's nonclinical, real life* that he or she (with support from loved ones) truly takes the first steps towards meaningful engagement. This sense of direct connection between one's own behavioral choices and one's nonclinical life, enjoyments, plans, and goals is *what engages patients to truly alter their behavior.*
Compassionate. Sincere. Personal. Engaging. Impactful. And for both patient and provider alike, *rewarding.*

For many patients, it is when a provider personally, compassionately links the individual's own health choices with that individual's nonclinical, real life that he or she (with support from loved ones) truly takes the first steps towards meaningful engagement.

Let's be brutally honest here. The overwhelming majority of physicians have neither the time (and many do not have the personality) to follow the guidelines in seeking successful patient engagement. Nor would this necessarily be considered a physician "working at the top of his or her license." Certainly physicians must play *a* role; and physicians must be highly supportive of other providers who implement this engagement strategy. And *administrators must allow providers the necessary time and resources* for successful engagement. But let's be clear: *nurses and health professionals must drive Patient Engagement* if we are to realize truly meaningful change in our society's health and healthcare system. If we fail to achieve large-scale Patient Engagement, then we will never move on to truly successful Patient Education. And we will never benefit from truly impactful Patient Empowerment.

In our motor vehicle analogy, the ultimate result of failing to expand Patient Engagement is millions of drivers and passengers traveling our roads with their seatbelts unbuckled.

> **◉ PEARL**
>
> It is the initial phase—Patient Engagement—that is so challenging because it is a result of numerous, complex factors and is encouraged by our society's acceptance that patients do not have to own their health.

Patients Are Not All the Same: Allocating Precious Patient Engagement Resources

By its very nature, Patient Engagement is often extremely time consuming and repetitive for the provider. Thus, Patient Engagement can be quite resource intensive, and the most critical resource required for successful Patient Engagement are nurses, allied health professionals, and physicians. Given the relative scarcity of these provider resources (particularly with *time* as the new, most valued COIN OF THE REALM), it is necessary to appreciate an important reality: *when it comes to allocation of human resources for Patient Engagement, not all patients are created equal.*

> When it comes to allocation of human resources for Patient Engagement, not all patients are created equal.

Shark Surfers

The muscular, tan surfer dude stands on the beach, his back to the waves. His cocky smile is aimed directly at the television camera, and he never looks directly at the female reporter to his right when answering her question.

"Yeah, Dude," he says to her (without looking away from the camera). "It was, like, *gnarly!*"

His left arm cradles his surfboard, which stands upright, tail planted in the warm sand, its narrow tip pointing toward the cloudless beach sky. A foot above where his arm disappears behind the board, an enormous chunk is missing, a massive, jagged, bite-shaped piece of fiberglass and Styrofoam removed in a single crunch.

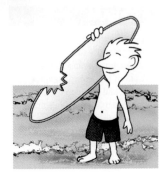

"Sure, Dude, *I know there are sharks out there,*" the teenaged Adonis says with swagger. "It's *their world* out there, Man. I know it. We all know it." Then he finally turns to the reporter, a big grin crossing his golden face. "But I love surfing, Dude. So if a shark kills me doing what I love . . . *so be it, Dude!*"

You've likely seen such a news interview from a beach in Australia or Hawaii or South Africa. A young man who is willing to die in the jaws of a shark to pursue the big wave. These are the *Shark Surfers.* Individuals who clearly recognize and appreciate that their personal choices, behaviors, and voluntary actions place them at significant risk, yet refuse to alter those behaviors.

There are Shark Surfers in the world of healthcare as well. Some swim for years with smaller, less immediately threatening sharks (smokers, obese individuals). Others swim with great whites (those who are noncompliant with life-sustaining medications, for example).

I was a resident on the *Red Surgical Service.* An apt name because surgeons on the Red Service inevitably saw a lot of blood during their 2-month rotation. The Red Service cared for the population of men and women whose alcoholism had eventually led to liver cirrhosis. Now, the healthy liver has the consistency of a big loofah sponge: not as soft as a standard kitchen sponge, but still compressible, with millions of tiny channels traveling throughout the three-dimensional structure. Channels that always allow the unimpeded flow of a massive volume of blood. But poisoned over decades by alcohol, that loofah turns into a brick. Liver cirrhosis. And the massive quantity of blood that needs to wind its way through the spongy liver becomes increasingly less able to do so as the liver hardens. Until at last, blood flow through the rock-hard liver virtually ceases to flow. Much like a plugged pipe, the obstructed blood backs up, swelling the veins of the spleen and stomach and esophagus (feeding tube) lying upstream.

One disastrous result for some cirrhotic patients is *bleeding esophageal varices,* a sudden, life-threatening, massive hemorrhage of blood from a vein in the esophagus that can no longer tolerate the chronically elevated pressure. I cannot describe the horror of someone bleeding in this fashion without being so graphic that you would close this book. Just believe me when I say,

The Walking Dead has nothing on this real-world, blood-pouring nightmare patient scenario.

We on the Red Service would work at lightning speed to try to save these hemorrhaging patients, transfusing in unit after unit of blood while racing to the operating room for a tour-de-force operation called a portacaval shunt. The details of this laborious, dangerous, multi-hour surgery aren't important for this story (and today, this procedure has been replaced by one performed by interventional radiologists). What is important is to understand that to survive *after* the operation (if lucky enough to survive the operation), a patient with a portacaval shunt *can only ingest a very, very small amount of dietary protein each day.* Too much protein and the patient will get loopy (demented) until the excess protein breakdown products are cleared from the body. Too, too much protein and the patient will fall into a coma (again, until the excess clears, which it does not always do). Too, too, too much protein and the patient simply dies.

Jerry had somehow survived prior to the emergency operation despite hemorrhaging out of his mouth faster than we could transfuse blood into him. Honestly, it was like the proverbial clown car at the circus, with red gush after red gush (where was it all coming from?). Then Jerry had somehow survived his many attempts to die right on the operating table. And after his portacaval shunt surgery, Jerry had somehow pulled through. And we were all thrilled when he was finally discharged home several weeks later. Jerry was a good guy—nice, bright, interactive, as was his very supportive, loving wife. Both Jerry and his wife were very clear in understanding about his postoperative dietary restrictions, particularly about the very real danger from eating too much protein over a short period of time. The dietician had counseled them both, and Jerry's wife held tightly to the list of acceptable and unacceptable foods.

For the first 4 months, Jerry did well. He stuck to his diet, he took his medications, he abstained from even a whiff of alcohol. He was a true success story and seemingly a man reborn.

Then it happened. Jerry was brought by ambulance to the ER. He was comatose. His wife was hysterical. We moved Jerry to the ICU, where we began to feverishly work to help his poisoned body recover.

"What happened?" I asked his exhausted wife as she sat in a chair next to his ICU bed.

"He had a bacon cheeseburger . . ." she told me, tears streaming down her cheeks.

Amazingly, Jerry was able to confirm exactly that several days later, when he awoke and his head eventually cleared.

"But . . . why?" I asked Jerry, confused. "Didn't you understand that a bacon cheeseburger is way too much protein for your damaged, surgically bypassed liver to deal with?"

"Sure," Jerry replied, without remorse. "It says 'Hamburger' right on the list that the dietician gave us. And I didn't think that adding bacon and cheese would make it any safer." He flashed a mischievous smile.

I just stared blankly at him, still trying to comprehend how two-plus-two equaled five. "Then," I repeated, *"why?"*

"C'mon doc," he said with a small smile. "What life is worth living without having a delicious, greasy bacon cheeseburger every now and then?"

Back then, I was too naïve a young physician to understand. Nor did I understand 2 months later when, again, Jerry arrived in a coma via ambulance, and again, we struggled to clear the toxins from his bloodstream as he lay in the ICU, his wife again sobbing in a chair next to his bed.

"He ate another bacon cheeseburger . . ." she whispered between sobs. "He *loves* bacon cheeseburgers."

"But . . ." I struggled, "but, he knows that bacon cheeseburgers are dangerous! He knows that eating them might kill him!"

Jerry's wife looked up at me, her crying momentarily halted. "Yes, Dr. Edelstein," she said stoically. "He knows." Then she paused. "He just loves bacon cheeseburgers."

Jerry's wife got it. I still did not, and it took me many more years and many more Jerrys before I finally (sort of) understood what she understood: *Jerry was a Shark Surfer.*

Jerry died during that third hospitalization from eating that second bacon cheeseburger. He died because he was unwilling to give up something he loved even though he clearly knew (had even experienced) the significant risk associated with his chosen behavior.

Some sharks come disguised as bacon cheeseburgers.

As it was in my case, it is often difficult for young (and even older) providers not only to understand Shark Surfers, but to actually identify their patient as a Shark Surfer.

Carol was a truly dedicated ER resident. I respected her passion for her patients as much as I did her significant knowledge of emergency medicine. Over the year that I had primary responsibilities for surgical evaluations and the provision of basic ER surgical care, we often worked long shifts together.

During that year, Carol and I must have cared for Eva at least half a dozen times. Carol likely saw Eva visit the ER more than that, as I only was involved in Eva's care when she needed a "shooter abscess" drained. A shooter abscess is a localized infection that develops at the site of a heroin injection, the result of an unclean needle, unclean skin, unclean heroin, or some combination of the three. Such collections of pus must be surgically drained before they make the patient seriously ill (often a minor procedure that can be performed in the ER). Eva was a heroin addict, and she supported her addiction through prostitution.

Now anyone who has spent significant time caring for patients in a busy, urban emergency room can tell you that everything you see on television hospital dramas is not always true. Eva was educated, pleasant, and often funny. She was, in fact, a pleasure to care for. And while my care was simply to surgically treat each new shooter abscess that brought Eva to the ER, Carol dedicated enormous amounts of her time and emotions on reforming Eva. It was always the same: you know that your choices are leading to these abscesses, and that you're at grave risk of getting AIDS or other sexually transmitted diseases. You know that there are programs available to help you with your addiction and to get you on a better path towards a clean life; etc.

And Eva was always engaged and very willing to hear this all again. Then she'd leave, only to return with another shooter abscess. And, eventually, with AIDs, from which she eventually (I learned later) died.

And Carol simply could not understand that . . . Eva was a Shark Surfer. Carol just couldn't see it. It simply didn't register.

We often don't see what's right in front of us. Especially if we don't want to see it or it fails to agree with our preconceived notions. Even experienced healthcare providers are often unable to truly recognize Shark Surfers for who they are, because the idea of Shark Surfers makes no sense to many healthcare providers. Shark Surfers knowingly act in ways that seem to provide little meaningful benefit while engendering significant risk. They are the antipatients, choosing a harmful pathway, forcing their loved ones to suffer emotionally, and for their providers to invest time and emotion and sweat into repeatedly "saving" them.

But if we are *willing to recognize them,* Shark Surfers tend to be easily identifiable for most experienced nurses, allied health professionals, and physicians (especially if they have a lifestyle and clinical history consistent with that of a Shark Surfer). Anyone actively involved in Patient Engagement today must not only appreciate but accept that there are Shark Surfers in our healthcare waters. And accept that *you can't save people who choose not to be saved.*

There are two more important points here, one grounded in reality and the other more philosophical. Let's start with reality. We simply do not have the resources (especially human) to continuously monitor our patient's lives to repeatedly intervene before they make their risk-associated choices. It's simply not possible. Even if I had been by Jerry's side every waking moment, the outcome might well have been the same. That is, *some people will always knowingly choose the risky behavior* (just think of the estimated *1 billion smokers worldwide*).[28]

> Anyone actively involved in Patient Engagement today must not only appreciate but accept that there are Shark Surfers in our healthcare waters. And accept that *you can't save people who choose not to be saved.*

Which leads us into the second, philosophical point: *is it appropriate for (let alone the responsibility of) the nurse, the physician, the therapist, or the dietician to turn the educated patient away from his or her chosen risk-associated behaviors?* Whose right and/or responsibility is it to force the young adult who believes himself immortal and who loves surfing more than life itself to abandon the waves because of what is likely swimming below? This philosophical debate is all-too-apparent today in the emotional battle over "Assisted Suicide." Should individuals with terminal diseases be allowed to choose a painless death "with dignity," or should society rigorously oppose such suicidal choice based on "moral grounds"? Should providers prolong every life for as long as possible, even when that "life" offers no hope of recovery to a level of any quality? Do any of us have the right to say with absolute certainty that Jerry was wrong, that life without bacon cheeseburgers is worth living, *for Jerry?* And if we do allow for such behavioral choices, *who should pay for the associated costs of care if the risks are realized?*

Whether or not your philosophical leaning supports the right of Shark Surfers to knowingly engage in health-destructive activities is less important than appreciating the reality of our healthcare system: our significant resource limitations (human and financial) render such philosophical debate somewhat moot. Trying to drive a true Shark Surfer to alter his or her risk-associated behaviors is simply too resource intensive and, ultimately, rarely successful. I base this conclusion after looking back over my decades of direct patient care during which I worked with more than a handful of Shark Surfers (whether or not I initially appreciated them as such). My conclusion continues with the belief that when caring for Shark Surfers, our provider responsibilities fall into three activities:

1. Make certain that to the best of their abilities and willingness, Shark Surfers and their loved ones are *educated and reeducated regarding the risks associated with their behavioral choices* (remember, Jerry was engaged and quite willing to be educated about his health risks; he just consciously refused to consistently reduce those risks), as Patient Education is a provider's responsibility.
2. If a Shark Surfer's voluntary behavior results in damage to their health, *always care for the Shark Surfer nonjudgmentally and to the best of your professional capabilities* (sometimes difficult, I can assure you, as you may often feel frustration with and even anger towards the patient).
3. Once (or if) the patient's health improves, again confirm that the Shark Surfer (and loved ones, if possible) clearly understands how their behavior led to their health damage, how you hope they'll consider avoiding the high-risk behavior moving forward, and that should they again hurt themselves through their behavioral choices, you will again do your very best to help them recover.

If you've identified a patient as a Shark Surfer, consider limiting the amount of time and energy you devote in repeatedly attempting to truly change his or her behavioral choices. I'm not being harsh or uncaring; the reality is that providers have only limited time and energy to devote to our entire patient population. It is a zero-sum game, so that the more time and energy devoted to Patient A, the less time and energy can be devoted to Patients B, C, and D. Shark

Surfers do not offer the provider the opportunity to get "the most bang for the buck." *On the Patient Engagement/ Education/Empowerment tree, Shark Surfers represent the highest hanging fruit.* What's most important (assuming that the Shark Surfer engages at all, which many actually do) is to focus on educating (and re-educating) the Shark Surfer and his or her loved ones, reinforcing the dangers associated with the behavior, that avoiding the behavior is a choice, and that should the Shark Surfer once again suffer a behavior-related health issue, you'll be there to help as best as you can. But spending hours of time and emotional capital trying to convince that sculpted, tan teenager to never again slip out over the waves on his surfboard . . . well that, my friends, is not the best allocation of limited resources.

> On the Patient Engagement/Education/ Empowerment tree, Shark Surfers represent the highest hanging fruit.

Credit Carders

Whereas Shark Surfers thankfully represent a true minority of patients (remember, just because a patient is *difficult* to engage does *not* mean that you have a true Shark Surfer on your hands), I suspect that a majority of our population falls into my second category: *Credit Carders.*

What's the subliminal message of every junk mail credit card pitch?

Own it now! Enjoy it now! Show it off now! (Pay for it later.)

Credit card companies both large and small attempt to tip the benefit-risk scale in their favor by implying that *you can realize immediate benefits/satisfaction/rewards (in exchange for a future, likely insignificant burden).*

In our healthcare world, the list of *Enjoy Now—Pay Later* examples could fill an ocean. To successfully engage Credit Carders, we must first understand the tactics that the Credit Carder uses subconsciously (or with partial or even complete awareness) to tip the benefit-risk scale in favor of poor health behaviors and decisions. Here are some common examples:

1. "I know that smoking causes cancer, but **smoking reduces my stress and keeps me from over-eating . . .**"
2. "I know that over-eating can lead to diabetes, but **eating reduces my stress and keeps me from smoking . . .**"

3. "I know that taking my blood pressure medicine is important, but **when I skip the pills, I'm not so tired . . .**"
4. "I know that colonoscopy can prevent colon cancer, but **I'm too busy to get screened . . .**"

These real-world statements exemplify the thematic tactics that Credit Carders (often empowered by family members using similar tactics) use to rationalize their behavioral choices and dismiss the health consequences associated with those decisions. Several tactics can be commonly identified:

Heavily Valuing the Immediate Benefit

Like the message in those endless credit card junk mailings, Credit Carders perceive the benefits of their behavioral choices as both real and immediate.

1. ". . . smoking *reduces my stress [now]* and *keeps me from over-eating [now]* . . ."
2. ". . . over-eating *reduces my stress [now]* and *keeps me from smoking [now]* . . ."
3. ". . . when I skip the pills, *I'm not so tired [now]*..."
4. ". . . I'm too busy *[so not undergoing cancer screening allows me to stick to my busy schedule now]* . . ."

Heavily Devaluing the Risk

At the same time that they lean heavily on the "benefit" side of the scale, Credit Carders also greatly reduce the weight pressing down on the "risk/burden" side. They do this through several approaches, often in combination:

- Credit Carders *disconnect any risk from themselves* from damaging their own health and life.
- They consider that risk as having *only the mere potential, often very low potential,* of ever being realized.
- They envision the risk as something vague rather than dangerously concrete.
  1. Rather than "I know that *my smoking* may mean that *I develop cancer,*" the Credit Carder distances *their chosen* behavior from the risk posed to their life: "I know that smoking causes cancer." Furthermore, in doing so, the cancer is something that may never occur, and even if it does occur, the impact is both far in the future and only vague in its impact.
  2. Instead of "I know that *my over-eating* may lead to *me getting diabetes,* which can lead to *my having a*

heart attack, kidney failure, and other serious health consequences," the Credit Carder waters down both the connection to self and the actual risk and damage that can result from their chosen actions: "I know that over-eating can lead to diabetes . . ."

3. The Credit Carder doesn't say, "I know that taking my prescription medications is critical to controlling my high blood pressure." Instead, the Credit Carder convinces themselves (and often their loved ones) that the absence of symptoms means that there is little or no risk in skipping the prescription medications.

4. "I know that colonoscopy can prevent colon cancer" is the Credit Carder's meaningless acknowledgement of the reality. This again completely distances Credit Carder from the risk (cancer) and from the potential and significant health and quality of life damage that colon cancer would have on his or her life. Any risk of colon cancer is framed as of low likelihood, far in the future, and entirely vague in its impact.

This emphasis on the immediacy and benefits of the voluntary behaviors; dissociation of the behavior-associated risks from self; and of characterization of the risks as unlikely, distant, and of vague consequence are some of the powerful psychological tricks that empower Credit Carders to continue their dangerous behaviors.

But *Credit Carders are not Shark Surfers.*

Shark surfers understand the risks associated with their behaviors and decisions and *consciously choose to accept those risks* rather than abandon their dangerous behaviors.

Credit Carders reduce or deny the risks associated with their behaviors and decisions, "giving themselves permission" to smoke, overeat, skip their medications, and avoid cancer screening.

This difference between the two patient categories is vitally important to appreciate because ultimately, unlike Shark Surfers, *Credit Carders can be engaged, educated, and empowered to change their behaviors and improve their health.*

> Ultimately, unlike Shark Surfers, Credit Carders can be engaged, educated, and empowered to change their behaviors and improve their health.

It is in understanding the psychological tricks that Credit Carders use on themselves that we can open the door to changing their behaviors. The nurse, pharmacist, dietician, physical therapist, physician who recognizes *the ways in which Credit Carders rationalize their poor health choices* is empowered to *successfully engage them.*

> It is in understanding the psychological tricks that Credit Carders use on themselves that we can open the door to changing their behaviors.

Engaging the Credit Carder

The steps to successful Patient Engagement have been outlined previously in this chapter ("The Basic Steps for A Provider to Initiate Meaningful Patient Engagement"). These steps, in the presented order, are your roadmap to engaging the Credit Carder. What is unique when engaging this group of patients (versus non–Credit Carders) is the need to *gently tear down their wall of psychological tricks to link their behavioral choices to the associated risks.* Remember, the Credit Carder *distances himself or herself from the risk* and consequences of the risk by *minimizing the likelihood* of the risk, placing any risk in the *way-distant future,* and by *significantly watering down the damage* resulting from risk realization (making the risk vague).

"So, Julia," Sara asked a moment after sitting down in the chair directly across from her patient in the outpatient exam room. "It was so nice meeting you a couple of weeks ago. I remember that you're 38 years old, and that you work at that big furniture store down on Market Street."

"I have to work," the overweight woman replied in a friendly tone. "I have an 11-year-old daughter."

"That's right," Sara said with a little laugh. "I remember. She sure sounds like a handful!"

"She sure is!" Julia said, her eyes sparkling. "She's smart. I want her to go to college. So I have to work."

Sara resisted her initial urge to now move into a conversation about her diabetic Credit Carder's behaviors. Instead, the provider continued to focus on the nonclinical aspects of her patient's life. "Seeing your daughter go to college is a wonderful goal. And it must be a great motivation to continue working."

Julia smiled and nodded.

Sara then asked, "Do you like working at the furniture store?"

"Yes, I do," Julia replied. "I'm the receptionist there. Everyone's really nice, and I've been there for 7 years already." She sat back in her chair and reflected on her words. "7 years already . . ."

"Wow," the provider said with a smile. "You've been working there for a long time. It must be a nice place to work. And you have a wonderful goal, being able to send your daughter to college."

Julia smiled. "Yes. I never went to college. I had to work. But I want her to experience college, and then she'll be able to choose what she wants to do."

"That will be wonderful," Sara said with a nod. "You seem like a great mother."

Julia's face expressed a mixture of embarrassment and pride.

Sara sensed that now the time might be right. "So," she maneuvered gently. "What would happen if you missed work? I mean, if you got really sick and couldn't work for a long time . . . or ever again?"

Julia was quiet for a moment. "That would be really bad," she finally said. "I mean, I'm divorced, and my daughter's dad is entirely out of the picture. My job is the only thing supporting us."

Sara said nothing, allowing Julia to keep considering the question.

"But I've never been sick. Not *really* sick, I mean. I've never missed more than a couple of days of work. You know, for the flu and stuff."

"Well, that's good," Sara said with a supportive nod. Then she leaned forward and took Julia's hands in her own. "Now, you know you have diabetes."

Julia barely nodded.

"And if your blood sugar isn't controlled, diabetes can get you really sick."

Again, a quiet nod.

"But *here's the good news,*" Sara said positively.

Julia looked into her provider's eyes.

"*Together,* I am confident that we can keep you healthy, and working, and caring for that little girl." The provider paused for a moment.

"At your last visit, and again today, your blood sugar is higher than we want it to be."

Again, a quiet nod of affirmation.

"Julia," Sara said while gently squeezing her patient's hands, "It's nothing to be ashamed of. It's simply an opportunity for us *together* to get your blood sugar under control. If we do that, and *together* I am certain we can, then we're doing something important. We're *keeping you healthy* so that you can continue being a great mother, continue working, and continue supporting your goal of sending your daughter to college. *Together* we can do these great things."

Sara smiled warmly. Julia let out a sigh of relief and returned the smile.

"Listen," Sara said, releasing Julia's hands. "Let's go over to the computer so we can learn *together* about a couple of simple but important things that you can easily do to control your blood sugar . . ."

Sitting side by side in front of the monitor, the provider and patient reviewed and discussed blood glucose monitoring, medication usage, and the role of hemoglobin A1c. A little later, Sara introduced her patient to a dietician, who together with Julia formulated a dietary plan to better control Julia's blood sugar levels.

And Julia returned to speak with Sara and the dietician 4 weeks later.

All right . . . this is a best-case scenario example. Not many conversations with Credit Carders go as easily as this, following a movie script. But you get the idea. The most successful approach to engaging a Credit Carder is through *personalization*. Personalization, as the word implies, requires *human-to-human interaction*. It is not a technology-based healthcare process. It requires the commitment of one or more compassionate care providers, but *it depends as well on healthcare administrators and leaders who appreciate that providers must be allowed adequate time* to get to know the patient and the patient's loved ones. No one "opens up" to a physical therapist or a Certified Diabetic Educator or a genetic counselor or a dietician who is obviously in a rush to get on with their other duties. And for the healthcare administrator, *there is significant* return on investment (ROI) if care providers are allowed the time to successfully engage Credit Carders.

The most successful approach to engaging a Credit Carder is through *personalization.*

It is of great value to include family members (particularly spouses and children), as well as friends and spiritual advisors (when appropriate), during the personalization process, as these individuals have both *a vested interest in the Credit Carder remaining healthy* as well as *far more frequent opportunities to advance the health ownership message.* Care providers must demonstrate sincere interest, compassion, and the patience (time) to get to know the patient, to connect with the patient and patient's loved ones on a truly personal level. Understanding just a bit about the Credit Carder's life, family, routine, plans, and even dreams provides a caregiver with targets at which to aim when moving to the next phase: *connecting the Credit Carder's voluntary behaviors in a positive way with meaningful risk reduction specific to the patient's life.* The care provider must address the tactics used by the Credit Carder to deflect responsibility and risk:

- Gain agreement that avoiding *very real risks* will have the *very positive effect* of reducing the likelihood of the patient himself or herself suffering the *concrete, negative consequences* which would clearly *interfere with specific favorable aspects of the patient's life* and plans.
- *Positively* emphasize that together with you and other providers, the patient can clearly *choose some well-defined behaviors and actions* that will lead to this *positive* risk reduction and *positive* protection of activities they enjoy currently and are looking forward to in their future.

A couple of points here. In our example, Sara wisely didn't "jump the gun" and begin discussing how type 2 diabetic Julia should *lose weight.* That should be a discussion *in the future,* but attempting to initiate a Credit Carder by first focusing on an enormously challenging goal (weight loss, complete smoking cessation, daily 30 minutes of exercise, etc.) often derails the train before it even leaves the station; that is, by *first* focusing on losing weight, Sara would likely have immediately lost any realistic opportunity to initially engage Julia. Rather, Sara chose to start with the immediate clinical challenge and risk and to focus on something with the potential to immediately deliver favorable results and positive reinforcement of Julia's behavior: improving Julia's blood sugar levels. By linking the opportunity to *together* better control her blood glucose levels with *positives* in Julia's life (continued good health, allowing her to work) and in Julia's future goals (earning money to send her daughter to college), Sara positively empowered Julia to engage (and not alone) in her own health and healthcare.

As Julia achieves success in controlling her blood glucose levels (even if at first that success is intermittent), Sara (and Julia's friends) can positively reinforce her healthy behaviors. In time, Sara (with the assistance of a dietician and exercise counselor) will likely be able to move into the next phase of Julia's engagement: realistically paced, incremental weight loss, again linking Julia's behavioral choices with positive outcomes specific to her life and goals.

It is of great value to include family members (particularly spouses and children), as well as friends and spiritual advisors (when appropriate), during the personalization process.

Nor is personalization always a long, laborious process. You must use your people skills and instincts to determine when your interaction with your Credit Carder has reached the appropriate point to turn the conversation towards the clinical situation and behavioral choices. In some cases, "the right time" may come along soon after first speaking with the patient. At other times, the opportunity to meaningfully engage the patient may only arise after several interactions. Learn from your successes and from your failures and trust your interpersonal skills (those same skills that led you into a career as a care provider). Most often, Credit Carders need to be reengaged over and over again (by providers, family, friends). Fortunately, once that personal understanding and connection between provider and patient have been established, revisiting engagement is both easier and faster for all involved (like riding a bike). Finally, opportunities to engage Credit Carders often present themselves in the ambulatory (even home) setting. And while engagement can be initiated or reinforced in the hospital, often by then, the Credit Carder's protective wall of dissociation between their behaviors and any vague, future, low potential risk has been shattered, as they've suffered some health event that has landed them in the hospital (there's nothing like lung cancer to make the behavior-associated risks of smoking suddenly concrete and real). In other words, for many Credit Carders, hospitalization represents the end result of failed Patient Engagement.

And remember, successful engagement is much more likely if the Credit Carder feels *part of a team*. Thus, again,

I cannot overstate the importance of engaging spouses, children, and friends in this process, as they allow for constant positive behavioral reinforcement and they are deeply invested in improving and protecting their loved one's health. The Credit Carder must feel that one or more providers is also actively "in their corner" as they strive to change their behaviors. Don't "bite off more than you can chew;" rather, ensure that the plan for behavioral change is *iterative and incremental,* beginning with smaller, realistically achievable goals that allow for success and the building of patient confidence. Don't let set-backs derail the process, but simply regroup and continue, *together.* "Let's aim at getting half of your blood sugar levels within the healthy range this week." If successful, increase the goal for the following week. If unsuccessful, *together,* and *as positively as possible,* analyze the sources of the failure and create a modified game plan for the next week.

It's all about personalization: positively connecting behavioral choices to the protection of current and future life activities that have deep, personal meaning for the patient.

Listen to any credible financial advisor and they'll tell you to *always pay off your monthly credit card bill* to avoid the massive interest costs, to use credit sparingly, and to only buy what you can truly afford. The same holds true in healthcare. Only when patients abandon their Credit Carder persona can they truly engage, become educated and empowered, and find their pathway to better health.

Different Drummers

I was a surgical fellow in freezing Minneapolis. On that particular day, I had just completed a colonoscopy (fiberoptic visualization of the large intestine) on an elderly man who was experiencing abdominal pain. The colonoscopy had identified a large colon cancer, and I was preparing to speak with the patient, his wife, and his two daughters about the tumor I had found, its implications, and his treatment options.

The man was Hmong[29] (the Hmong are refugees from Southeast Asia who were forced to flee their homeland after some assisted the United States during the Vietnam War). While he did not speak any English (and I speak no Hmong), I had requested that a hospital Hmong translator join us. (Minnesota has a large enough Hmong population[30] that Hmong translators are common in the hospitals.) The man's daughters, however, assured me that their English was strong enough to translate my words to their parents (and it appeared to be the case), but given that the hospital translator had already arrived, I asked her to stay just in case any medical terms or concepts were too difficult for the patient's two daughters to translate into their native tongue.

Still, it seemed that the translator was not needed. As I slowly explained that I had found a malignant tumor, what that cancer meant for their father, and my recommended approach to treatment (starting with surgery), the two girls seamlessly morphed my words and message into fluent Hmong.

When I was through, the girls assured me that neither their father nor mother had any questions (which I should have seen as the first "red flag," but being inexperienced, I only really appreciated this in retrospect), and they said that their father had agreed to have surgery as soon as possible.

As I smiled and nodded, I felt a light tug on my white coat. Turning my head, I saw that the hospital translator had a concerned look on her face as she quietly asked me to step away for a moment.

"What is it?" I asked with true curiosity, after she and I had stepped into a private room.

"The two girls told their father nothing that you said," she explained stoically.

I looked at her, dumbfounded. "What . . . what do you mean?"

"They told him that he had a 'small problem' in his intestine, and that you would 'easily fix it with a small operation.' And that the operation was 'entirely safe.'"

"But . . ." I stammered, "That's not what I said. And *what about the cancer?*"

"They never mentioned 'cancer.' They only said that you had found a 'small problem.'"

"And the risk of dying? And the risk of the surgery?" I asked, incredulously.

"No. They said nothing of these things."

"But . . . *why not?*" I asked her.

"We Hmong are not like you Americans. In our culture, we do not speak of such dangerous illnesses, or say that something done by the doctor could go wrong. It is our way to downplay dangers and risks when it concerns the health of our loved ones."

"But I must know that he knows the truth," I said. "That he knows he has cancer, and that he understands the risks of the surgery that he's agreeing to. It's not just the law, it's how we Americans practice medicine."

"Yes," she agreed. "That's why I suggest we return, and you allow me to translate it all again. As you have said it."

I nodded. Clearly, she had a better understanding of what to do here than I did.

"But," she continued, before we stepped out from our private room, "Let me first explain to the girls what we must do. They will be unhappy, but they will understand and allow it."

We headed down the hall. Before reaching the waiting family, the translator turned her head towards me and softly said, "And *he knows* that he has something very bad. *People always know.*"

When it comes to health and healthcare, many people "march to the beat of a different drum." There is no guarantee that what healthcare providers say, or how or why we say it, will be understood, make sense, or resonate with every patient, nor that every patient will be able to successfully communicate their questions, concerns, and thoughts with their providers. And unfortunately, the walls preventing us from actively engaging the majority of these *Different Drummers* are not always as easily scalable as language differences. In my (true) story, the major issue preventing successful patient engagement with my Hmong patient and his family was *not* our language difference (my naïve first impression), it was our *cultural* differences. And culture does not specifically imply American versus non-American, or one ethnic background versus another. When it comes to healthcare, the United States demonstrates numerous not-necessarily-so-obvious subcultures. For example, a common cultural challenge faced by providers every day (although they often fail to address it or even recognize it) is an *age-based subculture* in which provider communications with older Americans can be complex and challenging.[31] Even within this subpopulation, there are differing Different Drummer characteristics. Many of today's elderly, for instance, were raised to *never question a provider.* Thus these elderly Different Drummers simply allow their providers to make all healthcare decisions for them, never asking for explanations when they don't understand, and never objecting to the recommended plans. While this may seem like a perfect scenario for providers (after all, a dictatorship is the most efficient form of government), it is in reality a *poor situation for everyone* (including providers), as it is the ultimate example of *the unengaged patient driving down the value of healthcare.* Other older Different Drummers are easily overwhelmed by the information and explanations offered by their providers, as well as by the recommended health empowering technology, greatly limiting their successful engagement. And for still other elderly Different Drummers, differing psychological and societal challenges inhibit successful patient-provider communications.[32]

When it comes to health and healthcare, many people "march to the beat of a different drum." There is no guarantee that what healthcare providers say, or how or why we say it, will be understood, make sense, or resonate with every patient, or that every patient will be able to successfully communicate their questions, concerns, and thoughts with their providers.

Just as older age can result in a patient being a Different Drummer, *level of education* is another major, common variable impacting patient engagement. Simply put, a limited formal education inhibits the ability of some patients to be engaged if the provider does not recognize this barrier. While providers have adopted a large volume of language to address medical topics in "lay terms" (such as the use of "high blood pressure" rather than "hypertension," "heart attack" instead of "myocardial infarction," and explanatory phrases such as "breast cancer that has spread elsewhere in the body" in place of "metastatic adenocarcinoma of the breast"), in many cases of Different Drummers of limited education, simply modifying the words that providers use is not enough. Rather, the entire process of provider-patient communication must be modified to engage. Note that *this does not mean that less educated individuals cannot understand what their providers are saying.* It means that *providers must recognize this engagement barrier* and *respectfully communicate in terms and manner that allow the patient (and loved ones) to clearly understand and participate.*

Respectfully.

Educational, language, and cultural challenges independently and in combination together result in a major Different Drummer category that is catastrophic for patients and for our healthcare system: *low **health literacy.*** Defined by the ACA as "the degree to which an individual has the capacity to obtain, communicate, process, and understand basic health information and services to make appropriate health decisions,"[33] challenges with health literacy are found among Americans of all racial, ethnic, and even educational backgrounds. That said, poorer literacy is particularly associated with people of lesser education, those without health insurance, Medicare and Medicaid patients, and the elderly; yet even insured, educated, younger Americans often demonstrate limited health literacy.[34]

For the provider, therefore, *health literacy frequently represents a multifactorial obstacle to truly engaging the Different Drummer,* and you should never assume that just because you are caring for a bright, educated, younger patient, that man or woman truly understands the difference between "the colon" and "the large intestine" and "the large bowel" or between the "seasonal flu" and the "stomach flu." That is, education, intelligence, youth, ethnic background, wealth . . . none of these guarantees that your patient isn't a health literacy-impaired Different Drummer.

Nor is health literacy limited to written and/or spoken *words.* One form of health literacy that challenges many people is ***health numeracy,*** the inability to effectively understand, communicate, and process *numerical* health information, instructions, and recommendations. Even bright, educated patients are often unable to differentiate between a medication that is to be taken three times a day ("t.i.d." with no prescribed interval) and a medication to be taken "q8 hours" (strictly, every 8 hours).[35] Trust me . . . I've asked this question to rooms full of such individuals (including highly educated, successful CEOs) and have routinely been answered with silence and blank stares.

Health literacy challenges. Health numeracy challenges. Differing languages. Numerous cultures. Varying educational levels. All of these and other personal variables work independently and (often) in combination to create the largest pool of patients, Different Drummers. And *engaging Different Drummers is far more challenging* than engaging Shark Surfers (who often are happy to engage, just not interested in altering their behavior) or engaging Credit Carders (whose failure to engage is based on only a handful of common, addressable rationalizations).

Health literacy challenges. Health numeracy challenges. Differing languages. Numerous cultures. Varying educational levels. All of these and other personal variables work independently and (often) in combination to create the largest pool of patients, Different Drummers.

And here's one final important point: *even if you successfully address the challenges to engagement, that Different Drummer may then still turn out to be a Credit Carder or even a Shark Surfer!* If that's the case (and a Different Drummer who is also a Credit Carder is not uncommon), once you've knocked down the Different Drummer obstacles to communication, you then have to engage the Credit Carder or interact with the Shark Surfer who lies beneath.

> Even if you successfully address the obstacles to engagement, that Different Drummer may then still turn out to be a Credit Carder or even a Shark Surfer!

One can ask, "What's the real problem with an unengaged Different Drummer, as long as they follow my care recommendations?" For example, why didn't I just go ahead and operate on my Hmong patient with the colon cancer, given that he, his wife, and his daughters clearly would have allowed this (in fact, they preferred this to listening to an accurate translation of information regarding his cancer, prognosis, and treatment options). But what would my Hmong patient do if he developed a little difficulty breathing days after returning home following surgery? Or if he spiked a fever at home just days after his third round of chemotherapy? How would he know that these seemingly minor symptoms might represent life-threatening complications? Would he or his wife or his daughters immediately contact a provider, not appreciating their potential danger? Or would his family only take him to the ER once he had become so ill that he and his family could no longer deny that something was seriously wrong.

As we've pointed out many times in this book, *patients who fail to own their health are the main drivers of our poor-quality, high-cost healthcare.* And for the many reasons already noted, *Different Drummers fail to own their health.* We only have to look to the impact of literacy on patient health and our healthcare system to understand the damage done by unengaged Different Drummers. An individual's "functional literacy" can be measured by one of several instruments,[36] and numerous studies have clearly demonstrated the relationship between literacy, patient health, and the quality and cost of healthcare. Here's a small sampling of the dramatic conclusions from just a few literacy studies:

- *"Low literacy is associated with increased risk of hospitalizations and death among individuals with heart failure."*[37]
- *"Individuals with inadequate and marginal health literacy were more likely to die during follow-up than were those with adequate health literacy."*[38]
- *"Lower health literacy was associated with increased risk of death after hospitalization for acute heart failure."*[39]
- *"Health literacy and the risk of hospitalization"*[40] (Fig. 6.4)

Whether challenges are based on literacy, numeracy, language, culture, education, and/or some other personal characteristic, *Different Drummers are unable to actively engage in their own health and healthcare,* resulting in poorer health and lower value healthcare.

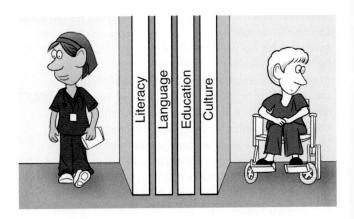

Just a few paragraphs ago, I said that "engaging Different Drummers is far more challenging than engaging Shark Surfers . . . or engaging Credit Carders." Well, yes . . . and *no.* The key to cracking the Different Drummer wall is to as quickly as possible determine those factors contributing to the communication and comprehension barriers. Sometimes the only real obstacle to successful Different Drummer engagement is just language, a fairly obvious barrier which is usually easily addressed with the help of a competent translator. In fact, often *addressing*

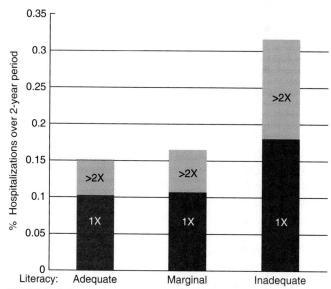

FIGURE 6.4 Health literacy chart. (Modified from Baker DW, Parker RM, Williams MV, et al. Health literacy and the risk of hospital admission. *J Gen Intern Med.* 1998;13[12]:791-798. http://dx.doi.org/10.1046/j.1525-1497.1998.00242.x.)

the Different Drummer challenge isn't the hard part; it's *identifying* the barriers that can be difficult. As my Hmong patient experience demonstrated, unlike language issues, recognizing cultural obstacles to true Different Drummer engagement is not always obvious. The same frequently holds true for appreciating literacy and numeracy obstacles to engagement (whereas once identified, and given adequate time and assistance, a provider can respectfully modify his or her communication and successfully engage the Different Drummer).

> Often *addressing* the Different Drummer challenge isn't the hard part; it's *identifying* the barriers that can be difficult.

It is arguably in engaging Different Drummers where physicians are often the least equipped for success. Not in dealing with language barriers, as today's hospitals routinely are staffed with a variety of language translators. But when patients don't obviously demonstrate cultural, literacy, numeracy, and/or educational impediments to engagement (as in the case of my Hmong family, and the situation with many elderly American patients), the overly busy physician may simply assume that he or she is communicating successfully and move on. This is not an excuse, it's just the reality (remember, for the provider, time is THE COIN OF THE REALM). So again, you can guess which providers are most suited to drive Different Drummer engagement: *nurses and allied health professionals.* These providers are best positioned to identify the barriers to engagement (never assuming that there is just one) based on their style and frequency of patient interactions. Once identified, the health professional or nurse must explore what lies underneath: Is the Different Drummer *ready* to be engaged? Is the Different Drummer also a *Credit Carder?* Or is this a Different Drummer who simply wishes to grab his or her surfboard and head back out into the shark-infested waters? How will the Different Drummer's *loved ones influence potential engagement* (for better, or as in the case of my Hmong patient's daughters, for worse)?

Nurses, therapists, dieticians, medical assistants, and other allied health professionals offer the greatest opportunity to successfully engage Different Drummers, and through the engagement of this enormous patient population, to dramatically improve America's health and healthcare.

> ● **PEARL**
>
> While there are many (often overlapping) reasons patients fail to engage, stratifying patients into *Shark Surfers, Credit Carders,* and *Different Drummers* provides a structural framework through which healthcare administrators can allocate resources and providers can understand the processes of engagement.

Putting It All Together

We still make the mistake of focusing too much attention on *changing the behavior of those who deliver healthcare* rather than on *those who play the much larger role in health and healthcare.*

> We still make the mistake of focusing too much attention on changing the behavior of those who deliver healthcare rather than on those who play the much larger role in health and healthcare.

Providers are the car manufacturers, the people who *provide* the seatbelts. Only *patients* (that is, everyone in the population) *can actually buckle up those seat belts.* Because of this overwhelming truth, nothing will more powerfully or sustainably lead America to improved health and higher value healthcare (both in terms of quality and cost) than Patient Engagement, Patient Education, and Patient Empowerment on a societal scale. This patient health ownership model must be our primary focus (and represents by far our greatest challenge) if we are to achieve meaningful healthcare reform. And who must be the primary leaders in this endeavor, both strategically and tactically?

Nurses and allied health professionals.

References

1. *Disease and Death in America: A Poor Bill of Health.* The Economist (online); 2013. http://www.economist.com/blogs/democracyinamerica/2013/07/disease-and-death-america.
2. Detsky A. *Why America Is Losing the Health Race.* The New Yorker (online); 2014. http://www.newyorker.com/tech/elements/why-america-is-losing-the-health-race.
3. Pampel FC, Krueger PM, Denney JT. Socioeconomic disparities in health behaviors. *Annu Rev Sociol.* 2010;36:349–370.
4. Rojas-Burke J. *Looking at the Relationship Between Scarcity, Unhealthy Behavior.* Assoc of Health Care Journalists (online); 2014. http://healthjournalism.org/blog/2014/07/looking-at-the-relationship-between-scarcity-unhealthy-behavior/.
5. Chetty R, Stepner M, Abraham S, et al. The association between income and life expectancy in the United States, 2001–2014. *JAMA.* 2016;315:1750–1766.
6. Tavernise S. *Disparity in Life Spans of the Rich and the Poor is Growing.* The New York Times (online); 2016. https://www.nytimes.com/2016/02/13/health/disparity-in-life-spans-of-the-rich-and-the-poor-is-growing.html?_r=0.
7. Zarroli J. *Life Expectancy Study: It's Not Just What You Make, It's Where You Live.* National Public Radio (online); 2016. http://www.npr.org/sections/thetwo-way/2016/04/11/473749157/its-not-just-what-you-make-its-where-you-live-says-study-on-life-expectancy.
8. *Economic Trends in Tobacco.* Centers for Disease Control and Prevention (online); 2017. https://www.cdc.gov/tobacco/data_statistics/fact_sheets/economics/econ_facts/index.htm.
9. *Study Estimates Medical Cost of Obesity May Be as High as $147 Billion Annually.* Centers for Disease Control and Prevention (online); 2009. https://www.cdc.gov/media/pressrel/2009/r090727.htm.
10. *Increase Expected in Medical Care Costs for COPD.* Centers for Disease Control and Prevention (online); 2014. https://www.cdc.gov/features/ds-copd-costs/.
11. *Safety Belts: Thousands of People Still Die Because They Didn't Buckle Up.* Insurance Institute for Highway Safety (online); 2017. http://www.iihs.org/iihs/topics/laws/safetybeltuse/mapbeltenforcement.
12. *Motor Vehicle Crash Deaths.* Centers for Disease Control and Prevention (online); 2016. https://www.cdc.gov/vitalsigns/motor-vehicle-safety/index.html.
13. Norris L. *I've heard that the government can't really enforce the penalty for not having health insurance. True?* HealthInsurance.org (online); 2016. https://www.healthinsurance.org/faqs/ive-heard-that-the-government-wont-really-be-able-to-enforce-the-penalty-for-not-having-health-insurance-is-this-true/.
14. McCarthy N. *Americans Visit Their Doctor 4 Times A Year. People In Japan Visit 13 Times A Year.* Forbes (online); 2014. https://www.forbes.com/sites/niallmccarthy/2014/09/04/americans-visit-their-doctor-4-times-a-year-people-in-japan-visit-13-times-a-year-infographic/#22e652dae347.

15. Brodwin E, Radovanovic D. *Here's How Many Minutes the Average Doctor Actually Spends with Each Patient.* Business Insider (online); 2016. http://www.businessinsider.com/how-long-is-average-doctors-visit-2016-4.

16. Japsen B. *For Every Hour with Patients, Doctors Spend Two Record-Keeping.* Forbes (online); 2016. https://www.forbes.com/sites/brucejapsen/2016/09/06/for-every-hour-with-patients-doctors-spend-two-record-keeping/#e5b97fe29501.

17. Mitchell RJ, Bates P. Measuring health-related productivity loss. *Popul Health Manage.* 2011;14:93–98.

18. Japsen B. *US Workforce Illness Costs $576B Annually From Sick Days To Workers Compensation.* Forbes (online); 2012. https://www.forbes.com/sites/brucejapsen/2012/09/12/u-s-workforce-illness-costs-576b-annually-from-sick-days-to-workers-compensation/#1d2a25335db0.

19. Alkire M. *Why an Aspirin Taken in a Hospital Can Cost Upwards of $25.* Healthcare Finance (online); 2012. http://www.healthcarefinancenews.com/blog/why-aspirin-taken-hospital-can-cost-upwards-25.

20. Graham J. *Obamacare's Individual Mandate Is Really Inefficient.* Forbes (online); 2017. https://www.forbes.com/sites/theapothecary/2017/01/20/obamacares-individual-mandate-is-really-inefficient/#746c6cc53ecb.

21. King R. *Obamacare Program Unfairly Penalizes Safety-Net Hospitals: Senators.* Washington Examiner (online); 2015. http://www.washingtonexaminer.com/obamacare-program-unfairly-penalizes-safety-net-hospitals-senators/article/2569567.

22. Serrie J. *More than 2,200 Hospitals Face Penalties under ObamaCare rules.* Fox News (online); 2012. http://www.foxnews.com/politics/2012/08/23/more-than-2200-hospitals-face-penalties-for-high-readmissions.html.

23. Markay L. *Study: Obamacare Penalizes Hospitals Serving Low-Income Medicare Patients.* The Washington Free Beacon (online); 2015. http://freebeacon.com/issues/study-obamacare-penalizes-hospitals-serving-low-income-medicare-patients/.

24. Eggen D. *Rick Perry Reverses Himself, Calls HPV Vaccine Mandate a 'Mistake'.* The Washington Post (online); 2011. https://www.washingtonpost.com/politics/rick-perry-reverses-himself-calls-hpv-vaccine-mandate-a-mistake/2011/08/16/gIQAM2azJJ_story.html?utm_term=.bfd1ea8a568e.

25. *HPV Vaccine: State Legislation and Statutes.* National Conference of State Legislatures (online); 2017. http://www.ncsl.org/research/health/hpv-vaccine-state-legislation-and-statutes.aspx.

26. High Blood Pressure Health Risk Calculator. American Heart Association/American Stroke *Association* (online); http://tools.bigbeelabs.com/aha/tools/hbp/

27. Stanik-Hutt, Newhouse RP, et al. The quality and effectiveness of care provided by nurse practitioners. *J Nurse Pract.* 2013;9:492–500.

28. Tobacco. World Health Organization (online) 2016; http://www.who.int/mediacentre/factsheets/fs339/en/

29. Hmong Culture. HmongCulture.net (online); http://www.hmongculture.net/hmong-people.

30. Hmong in Minnesota. Minnesota Historical Society (online); http://www.mnhs.org/hmong.
31. Williams SL, Haskard KB, DiMatteo MR. The therapeutic effects of the physician-older patient relationship: effective communication with vulnerable older patients. *Clin Interv Aging*. 2007;2:453–467.
32. Day T. About Medical Care for The Elderly. *National Care Planning Council* (online); https://www.longtermcarelink.net/eldercare/medical_care_issues.htm.
33. *What is Health Literacy?* Centers for Disease Control and Prevention (online); 2016. https://www.cdc.gov/healthliteracy/learn/.
34. *America's Health Literacy: Why We Need Accessible Health Information*. Department of Health and Human Services (online); 2008. https://health.gov/communication/literacy/issuebrief/.
35. *When is TID not q8h?* Public Health Resources (online); 2014. https://publichealthresources.blogspot.com/2014/03/when-is-tid-not-q8h.html.
36. Collins SA, Currie LM, Bakken S, et al. Health literacy screening instruments for ehealth applications: a systematic review. *J Biomed Inform*. 2012;45:598–607.
37. Wu JR, Holmes GM, DeWalt DA, et al. Low literacy. *J Gen Intern Med*. 2013;28:1174–1180.
38. Baker DW, Wolf MS, Feinglass J, et al. Health literacy and mortality among elderly persons. *Arch Intern Med*. 2007;167:1503–1509.
39. McNaughton CD, Cawthon C, et al. Health literacy and mortality: a cohort study of patients hospitalized for acute heart failure. *J Am Heart Assoc*. 2015;4:e00179.
40. Baker DW, Parker RM, Williams MV, et al. Health literacy and the risk of hospital admission. *J Gen Intern Med*. 1998;13:791–798.

CHAPTER 7

Clinical Decision Support

It is impossible to separate healthcare from politics for two simple reasons: first, every one of us will at some point become consumers (customers, if you prefer) in our nation's healthcare system (for most of us, more and more frequently as we age); second, healthcare spending represents a significant portion of our economic engine, impacting government coffers and our individual wallets alike. Just a quick perusal of the news headlines from the past several years through today reveals article after article reporting on the emotionally charged healthcare reform debate. Thus it was not surprising that many healthcare professionals viewed the Affordable Care Act's legislated implementation timeline for reform activities, programs, and penalties to be more reflective of political needs rather than of operational realities, because shifting close to 18% of the country's gross domestic product from our entrenched, traditional fee-for-service model to a starkly different value-based system cannot be rapidly achieved.

My own experience as a physician executive in a large, multistate **integrated delivery network (IDN)** mirrors that of the nurses, pharmacists, and other healthcare professional leaders with whom I have spoken over the last several years: following the passage of reform legislation in 2010, healthcare C-suites (executives) across America scrambled to understand just what the law and timelines and (especially) financial penalties meant for their healthcare systems, providers, and patients. All heard the loud (and getting louder) ticking of the reimbursement penalty clock, driving provider organizations (the punitive target of the legislation) to aggressively search for technologies offering solutions to the requirements and threats posed by the new reform law. Unfortunately, in their rush to comply with this accelerated paradigm shift in the healthcare delivery model, *many provider organizations failed to first allocate adequate time for the creation and development of sound strategies to successfully achieve and sustain value-based care.*

Following the passage of reform legislation in 2010, healthcare C-suites across America scrambled to understand just what the law and timelines and (especially) financial penalties meant for their healthcare systems, providers, and patients.

The adoption of electronic health record (EHR) systems is a dramatic example of this failure to "put the horse before the cart;" that is, to adequately develop a strategy prior to buying the tools. Driven by potential Meaningful Use[1] incentives and penalties, provider organizations raced to purchase EHRs, many without first defining their short- and long-term goals, understanding their resources, or recognizing how differing EHR systems would fit into their strategy. Thus, while the US **Office of the National Coordinator for Health Information Technology (ONC)** noted that "Hospital adoption of EHR systems more than tripled"[2] between 2009 (the year prior to the signing of the ACA) and 2012, by 2015, *60% of EHR purchases represented replacements of previously purchased EHRs.*[3]

What does it say when the majority of new EHRs are purchased t*o replace previously purchased, implemented, functioning EHR systems* purchased only a few years earlier?

It says that hundreds of millions of dollars have been wasted because we failed to first clearly understand our

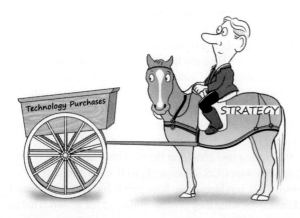

goals, inventory our resources, and appreciate the capabilities of the available technological solutions in our panic to avoid federally legislated reimbursement penalties. That is we put the "buy it" cart before the "strategic" horse.

If EHRs are the vehicle through which we will travel to higher value healthcare, then *current, credible, evidence-based information, knowledge, and guidelines* are the fuel that will power us to reach our goal. One of the many great things about the American economy is that if there is a profitable market, in a flash, there will be a product. Healthcare reform created a vast market desperate for current, credible, evidence-based technological solutions promising to drive high value healthcare, and consultants and health information technology (HIT) vendors began popping out of the ground like daisies. Their "solutions" to the demands, promises, and threats of healthcare reform were offered under a variety of labels, including Clinical Decision Support (CDS), **Reference Solutions,** and **Workflow Solutions.** (For the sake of simplicity, I'll use "Clinical Decision Support" or "CDS" to refer broadly to all such evidence-based healthcare information solutions.)

> If EHRs are the vehicle through which we will travel to higher value healthcare, then *current, credible, evidence-based information, knowledge, and guidelines* are the fuel that will power us.

What Are Clinical Decision Support Solutions?

While a detailed description of the dozens of types of CDS solutions is beyond the scope of this work, it is worth discussing some of the most prominent forms of CDS in use today (and tomorrow). The majority of CDS solutions are designed to integrate within the EHR. However, with so many EHRs being replaced within the United States, and given that EHRs are far from common in healthcare facilities outside the United States, CDS integration is often not possible. Thus many of today's CDS solutions can also function independently (utilized as independent websites or applications on your computer or mobile device), and most allow for information to be printed if desired.

A recurring and annoying theme within healthcare reform is apparent with CDS solutions as well: even similarly labeled CDS products often have subtle (or even significant) differences in what they profess to do and for whom. That is, no two **"Care Plans"** or "Reference Solutions" are the same. So keeping that in mind, what follows are a few generalized descriptions of commonly available and utilized CDS solutions.

Reference Solutions

Traveling from your hometown to Vegas for the weekend? One of the first things you'll likely do is go online to Orbitz. com or some other airline reference site to see what flights are available that fit your traveling plans. Want to better understand how customers like (or don't like) that new smartphone you're thinking about buying? Go online to check out customer reviews. TripAdvisor.com, AngiesList. com, and hundreds additional online reference sites have become part and parcel of our daily lives, assisting us when we need information. Electronic reference tools have not only replaced print (do you still have an encyclopedia in your den, a dictionary on your desk, or a thick phonebook in your kitchen?), they have expanded into thousands of spaces previously inaccessible in the past print-only age.

When it comes to health issues, the number of e-reference sites seems infinite (medical information websites run by healthcare systems, hospitals, individual practices, professional societies, nonprofits, and patient groups, to name only a few). There are so many to choose from when we need health and healthcare information! But there is very real danger lurking in many of these self-proclaimed credible reference sites because *not all healthcare reference "information" is equal.* Or even accurate. And incorporating erroneous information into your patient care can clearly threaten the quality (and cost) of that care. Thus it is critical that nurses, allied health professionals, doctors, pharmacists, and other providers only seek knowledge from *credible reference sites founded in current, evidence-based information.*

> It is critical that nurses, allied health professionals, doctors, pharmacists, and other providers only seek knowledge from *credible reference sites founded in current, evidence-based information.*

Yet ask allied health professionals where they get their healthcare reference information, and they'll frequently reply, "Wikipedia," or some other analogous general, anyone-can-input-information site. Why? *It's free and it's fast.*

Fair enough. Wikipedia (and similar sites) are free and are fast. However, *they are also filled with errors that pose real dangers to the practice of healthcare and to our patients.* In a review of the 10 most costly healthcare conditions in the United States, researchers found that "Most Wikipedia articles contain many errors when checked against standard peer-reviewed sources." The authors concluded that "Caution should be used when using Wikipedia to answer questions regarding patient care."[4]

So Wikipedia and other reference sites are free and fast and *inaccurate and potentially dangerous when used to guide health and healthcare decisions.*

> Wikipedia and other reference sites are free and fast and inaccurate and potentially dangerous when used to guide health and healthcare decisions.

Here is the staggering numerical reality: *every year, over 2.5 million new scientific papers are published* in over 2800 English language and over 6400 non–English language journals,[5] and the number is growing. Add this to *the 25 million available original scientific publications* (up to 50 million[6] based on how far back in history you're willing to go), and the challenge for any individual provider and patient becomes strikingly clear. Simply evaluating all of these millions of articles published by individual clinicians, researchers, professional societies, and others; then selecting those most critical to patient care; and finally consistently transferring all of this into electronic forms and for use by providers in the appropriate CDS solutions is both enormously time-consuming and costly. In other words, *quality current, credible, evidence-based Reference Solutions are not free.*

But as the old saying accurately states, *you get what you pay for.* And while it's one thing to utilize inaccurate information when driving to an unfamiliar restaurant, it's quite another thing to use erroneous information when providing emergent care for an obese diabetic with moderate renal failure who is suffering from acute heart failure. The ultimate return on investment (ROI) in terms of both safe, high-quality patient care and cost-efficient patient care is only realized when using Reference Solutions developed by expert commercial vendors possessing both broad and deep experience in regularly finding, evaluating, grading, and updating millions of research and clinical reports annually and placing these into formats which most easily drive high value patient care.

And, like Wikipedia, the most user-friendly Reference Solutions allow the allied health professional, nurse, doctor, patient, or other provider to search under any number of terms and rapidly find what they're looking for. They are, in effect, like Google or Yahoo. Enter "decub," and you should be offered numerous topics relating to "decubitus ulcers." Click on the topic that most fits your information

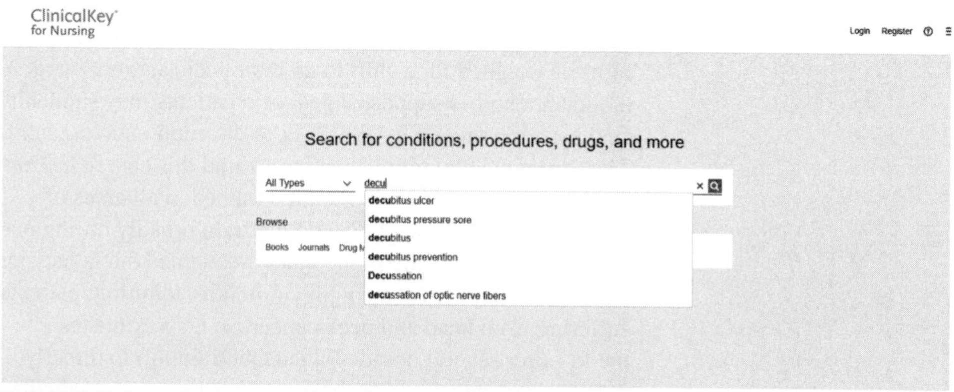

FIGURE 7.1 A Nursing-Specific Reference Solution Landing Page. Note: the author is employed by Elsevier, whose Nursing Reference solution is depicted here.

needs, and you should be immediately presented with journal articles, books and book chapters, guidelines, videos, high-definition images, and other formats presenting current, credible, evidence-based information on your selected topic. Available on mobile devices, the best Reference Solutions empower patient care at the bedside, in the home, or at any traditional or nontraditional care site. But the most powerful Reference Solutions also allow for deep dives into complex topics, providing clinicians with greater understanding of healthcare topics should they desire such knowledge and providing support for those who themselves are participating in research activities.

In the end, the best care providers are supported by current, credible, evidence-based information. That information comes from high-value Reference Solutions (Fig. 7.1) that, yes, cost money.

Clinical Skills Solutions

As hospitals and ambulatory centers desperately search for ways to reduce costs, it is no surprise that the first area they routinely target is what is often the greatest source of expense: staff salaries and wages. That is, management frequently begins cost-cutting discussions with "Are there any staff positions that we can eliminate?" Thus one expense reduction approach that is becoming more and more common is reducing the overall number of nurses and allied health professionals actively working within a care facility at any one time. So how do such facilities compensate for reduced numbers of caregivers? They assign the remaining nurses and allied health professionals to care delivery areas across the hospital, often placing these providers in less familiar health delivery scenarios. Thus a ward nurse who has spent years caring for internal medicine patients may suddenly find himself assigned for a shift to an orthopedic surgery ward. A dietician who has supported pediatric patients may suddenly find herself assigned for the week to the adult oncology unit. The (questionable) rationalization behind this cost reduction model is that providers at one time trained in all areas of care. Of course, those of us who did train broadly during our early educational years immediately recognize the fallacy in this logic. That I spent a couple of months admitting patients suffering from head and neck cancers in no way makes me fit (after several decades since that training) to directly care for such patients. For that reassigned internal medicine nurse, it may similarly have been years since she cared for a patient with a lower extremity external fixation device. The dietician may also not have studied any of the current guidelines for care of the adult metastatic breast cancer patient with cachexia. In a nutshell, for many providers who suddenly find themselves caring for patients suffering from less familiar conditions, this responsibility can be frightening (and dangerous for the patients).

That's where Clinical Skills solutions come in. Designed to support nurses and allied health professionals working in less familiar care situations (including in facilities which are new to the provider), these text and video solutions offer short, clear, and accurate instructions on delivering current, credible care. Don't remember how to change the dressing on a PICC line? Search your Skills solution and find a half-page telling you exactly what dressings and equipment you'll need. Click on the short video and watch a provider like you performing exactly the task you need to perform.

Clinical Skills (Fig. 7.2) are extremely powerful in ensuring that providers practicing in less familiar care situations are able to provide the best care to their patients.

Order Sets

Virtually every patient care activity (even the mundane) requires a documented physician order. What this patient can and cannot eat; any of that patient's activities that are limited or require assistance; this patient's known allergies; the administration (including dose, route, and frequency) of every single medication to that patient; every one of the many diagnostic tests (such as blood work and imaging studies) that a patient is to undergo; instructions for assessing each patient's vital signs; directions for the administration of intravenous (IV) fluids; resuscitation in the event of

Nutrition and Fluids
Taking Aspiration Precautions ▼

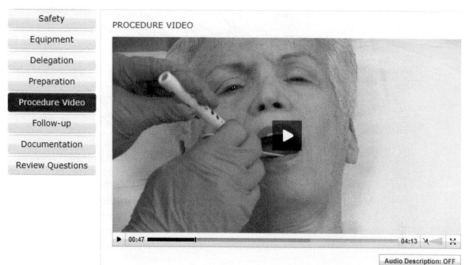

FIGURE 7.2 Clinical Skills solutions use text, animation, and video to guide the provider through thousands of routine care activities. *Note: the author is employed by Elsevier, whose Clinical Skills solution is depicted here.* (Image from Mosby: *Mosby's Nursing Video Skills: Student Online Version,* 4e, St. Louis, 2014, Mosby.)

cardiopulmonary arrest; *everything.* Orders are created *(initiated)* by physicians, but *they are used by all provider types* to guide all patient care activities. That said, the variability in legibility of hand-written physician orders (the traditional physician order format) has been the source of enormous patient safety problems. That's because pharmacy technicians, phlebotomists, respiratory therapists, nurses, radiology technicians, occupational therapists, and other providers often struggle to decipher what the physician has written in rushed, sloppy lettering[8,9,10] (Fig. 7.3).

But easily addressing the dangers of poorly written orders requires only a Computerized Provider Order Entry (CPOE) system (in fact, simply typing orders in Microsoft Word or a similar text program can avoid many order-related medical errors). But *Order Set solutions are so much more than clearly typed orders.* Order Sets can *improve patient care by offering current, credible, evidence-based, patient-specific guidance* to providers, even information about which the provider is entirely unaware. Traditionally, the physician wrote orders based on professional training and experience, memorizing what orders were needed for patients suffering from specific conditions and following specific tests and procedures. Again, the list of orders was lengthy,

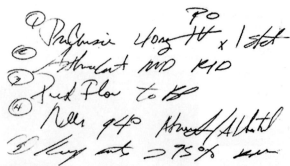

FIGURE 7.3 Real example of hand-written physician orders, clearly demonstrating the challenge for those providers required to follow these orders and the dangers posed to patients.[7] Courtesy of Kris Mastrangelo, OTR/L, MBA, LNHA President & CEO. Medicare Documentation for the Rehabilitation Patient. Harmony Healthcare International, Inc. (online presentation) 2014; https://www.slideshare.net/HarmonyHealthcareInternational/medicare-documentation-for-the-rehabilitation-patient-evidence-of-progress.

including such things as diet; physical activities; lab tests; imaging studies; respiratory care; allergy warnings; IVs; all medications; physical, occupational, respiratory, speech, and other therapy needs; etc. But this left the physician to rely on his or her own knowledge and memory, which often did not include newer (current) information (as few providers have the time to regularly keep current with more than a handful of patient conditions). *Enter Order Set solutions!* Created by interprofessional teams of experts (therapists, nurses, dieticians, pharmacists, radiographers, doctors, etc.) who constantly review the most recent evidence regarding care for specific patient scenarios, Order Sets offer current, credible, evidence-based guidance to the ordering physician (and, thus, the provider team) in any setting across the care continuum. Additionally, Order Sets are incredibly powerful, because they can push current best practice information which is unfamiliar to the providers as "recommended orders." For example, a physician who is unaware that a genetic test is both available and recommended for a younger patient with a right-sided colon cancer will be presented with a recommendation to order the appropriate genetic blood test; in addition, the Order Set (Fig. 7.4) can be linked to a Reference Solution, allowing the physician (or any provider) to learn much more about both the genetic test and the genetic disorder from which the patient may be suffering, all with a simple click of the mouse. All of this power to drive high-quality, cost-efficient patient care makes Order Set solutions far more than just the answer to illegible handwriting.

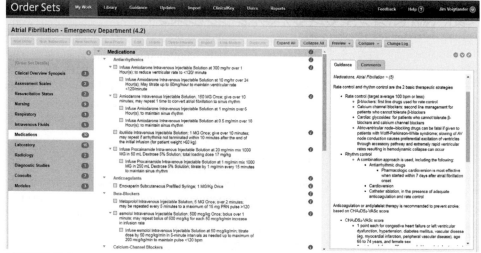

FIGURE 7.4 Order Set solutions can be condition and patient scenario-specific, empowering providers through current, credible, evidence-based guidelines. *Note: the author is employed by Elsevier, whose Order Set solution is depicted here.*

Drug Information Solutions

Drug Information solutions are just what they sound like they are: electronic databases offering everything a provider working in clinical pharmacology needs to know to support high value patient care. Given the significant role that medication errors play in preventable medical errors,[11] having rapid access to correct dosing, adverse reactions, contraindications, use in pregnancy and pediatrics, adjustments for liver or renal impairment, toxicity, comparable medicines, even costs (that is, to voluminous collections of pharmaceutical information) empowers pharmacists, pharmacy health professionals, and other providers in rapidly finding specific answers to specific medication-related questions. And as with all CDS solutions, it is critical that the information provided in Drug Information solutions is kept current, comes from credible sources, and is evidence-based.

Care Plans

Care Plans represent a major step forward in CDS solutions by offering current, credible, evidence-based *interprofessional care delivery plans which guide consistent patient care across the care continuum.* In effect, Care Plans seek to get all of a specific patient's providers at all points of care delivery "on the same page." Thus Care Plans focus on increasing patient safety and elevating quality (and, as a result, improving cost efficiency) associated with transitions in patient care (such as occur with patient transfer from ICU to ward, from hospital to SNF (skilled nursing facility), and even from hospital shift to shift). Given that challenges in provider-to-provider communication have been linked to significant patient safety and cost-of-care issues, Care Plans offer an approach to improving multiple provider, multisetting, patient-specific care.[12,13,14]

Clinical Pathways

The next generation of CDS solutions is the clinical pathway. At present, the definition of "Clinical Pathways" is more of a moving target than that of any other CDS solution. In other words, "Clinical Pathways" means different things (often very different) to different healthcare stakeholders. Even the category is not uniformly accepted, as other terms, such as "Clinical Maps" and "Care Pathways," are also frequently used.

Still, in trying to find common themes among the more frequently used definition, Clinical Pathways are sort of *Care Plans on steroids.* That is, they are *patient-centric, interprofessional,* and for use by providers across all care settings. However, Clinical Pathways offer even more than current, credible, evidence-based guidance. Clinical Pathways developers are utilizing *machine learning* ("the science of getting computers to act without being explicitly programmed")[15] and even *artificial intelligence* within these CDS solutions. When (not "if") successful, Clinical Pathways will be almost Star Trek–like in nature, offering certain evidence-based recommendations over others based on numerous, varied clinically specific, patient-specific, and scenario-specific factors. Think of the prostate cancer patient: there are so many crucial clinical factors (disease stage, Gleason score, comorbidities, etc.), relevant personal characteristics (functional age, sexual activity level, acceptability of urinary incontinence, etc.), and socio-economic considerations (regular transportation to and from multiple radiation therapy sessions, etc.) that must be considered when recommending the most appropriate, patient-specific treatment option. A Clinical Pathways solution that utilizes machine learning or artificial intelligence to weigh so many varying, seemingly unrelated factors will empower providers of all types in developing patient-specific recommendations. Mr. Spock would certainly support such a logical approach to patient care, although Dr. McCoy would no doubt be skeptical (yes, I am dating myself as a fan of the original Star Trek series).

Today, the first of these amazing Clinical Pathways solutions are entering the marketplace, empowering nurses, allied health professionals, physicians, and patients in achieving safer, more cost-efficient, patient-specific healthcare.

The Initial Disappointment in Implemented Clinical Decision Support

For many provider organizations, the appearance of CDS vendors offering a variety of health information technology (HIT) products to guide them safely through the healthcare reform gauntlet represented the proverbial cavalry coming over the hill. And so hospitals and healthcare systems and provider organizations bought and bought and bought. But just as with EHRs, many buyers purchased a variety of costly CDS solutions without first forming a clear CDS strategy. And again, spending without a strategy was a recipe for failure.[16,17,18]

I'm so excited! It's time to buy a new car! I really like the engine in the Porsche Turbo Carrera. So I buy it. *Just the engine,* mind you. Because I really like the Porsche engine, but I prefer the chassis of the Ford F-150 pick-up truck. So I buy one. *Just the chassis.* Now for the seats, for the entire interior of my awesome new vehicle, I look no further than the Mercedes S550. Plush, leather seats (with seat warmers!), a terrific GPS system, power mirrors, everything at the touch of a button. And when it comes to tires, you can't be too safe. So I'm going with the tires they use on Boeing 757 jets. You know: those big, thick, rubber jet tires. Eight of them! Now just add a windshield from an urban police SWAT assault vehicle to protect me from any flying gravel and other projectiles, and I'm all set. Time to "integrate" all of the "best in class" pieces together into the world's greatest car!

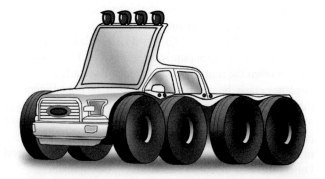

What's my point here (other than that I should never design cars)? This is exactly how too many US hospitals and healthcare networks went about building their CDS "integrated systems." Provider organization leaders feared that the rapidly approaching reimbursement penalties would sink them, and so they reached out for anything that promised to protect their finances. Without first truly understanding and defining their strategic value improvement goals, without thoroughly recognizing their vulnerabilities and gaps, without honestly appreciating their financial and human resource limitations and needs, *without carefully forming a clear and realistic and detailed strategy for success,* healthcare stakeholders forked over enormous amounts of money to CDS vendors. And just as I built my imaginary car, provider organizations bought Nursing Reference Solutions from Vendor A, Drug Information Solutions from Vendor B, Patient Engagement Solutions from Vendor C, Clinical Skills from Vendor D, Ambulatory Order Sets from Vendor E (but Inpatient Order Sets from Vendor F), Care Plans from Vendor G, and an EHR from Vendor H (an EHR which did not support integration of the CDS solutions purchased from Vendors A through G).

Get the (dysfunctional) picture?

In their panic and confusion over the complexity of legislated value-based reimbursement, many provider organizations used the "shotgun approach" in purchasing CDS solutions. The lack of coordination between clinical leaders in purchasing decisions only exaggerated the failure of this approach. Thus, even if nursing leaders provided input into CDS nursing solution purchases, these decisions were often made in isolation, without consultation from the pharmacists and physical therapists and case managers who were simultaneously evaluating CDS solutions specific to their fields (again, resulting in something akin to my car). The result is that today, many care providers must function in a world absent of a well-defined and communicated CDS strategy, working with CDS solutions which are neither technologically or (more importantly) clinically integrated.

But the challenges and failure of CDS solutions to improve healthcare are far from purely technological. Just as pilot error is often the root cause when technologically advanced airplanes crash, human behavior is often the impediment to the success of CDS in improving healthcare. Many nurses and allied health professionals complain that although potentially beneficial, EHRs and CDS solutions slow them down so much that the benefits of use are not worth the time required. Others feel that they don't need patient care guidance,

PEARL

As with initial EHR purchases and adoption, many healthcare facilities and organizations are only recently recognizing that the integration of CDS solutions without first forming a clear strategy based on honest evaluation of goals and resources will fail to significantly improve the value of delivered care.

confident (or arrogant) in their training and experience. What makes CDS utilization even more challenging is that *we don't even have concrete metrics by which to determine if an individual healthcare provider is appropriately using CDS solutions to support high value care delivery:*

> Question #1: Would you feel comfortable being cared for by a respiratory therapist who searches for current, credible, evidence-based care information *100 times each day?*

> Answer: Of course not, as this suggests that the respiratory therapist is not adequately trained and lacks adequate experience to care for patients.

> Question #2: Would you feel comfortable being cared for by a critical care nurse who searches for current, credible, evidence-based care information *once every 7 years?*

> Answer: Of course not, as this suggests that the critical care nurse is not keeping current on changes defining the best patient care.

The fact is, *no one can clearly say what appropriate usage of CDS solutions is for any individual provider.* Therefore, even tracking "usage" (which we do) and analyzing "usage" (which we do) does not necessarily clearly identify which providers are appropriately incorporating CDS solutions into their patient care workflow. And even those who routinely do access CDS solutions often complain of problems such as "alert fatigue,"[19] while other regular users frequently ignore the presented CDS guidance.[20]

Such individual provider challenges are compounded by systematic challenges, such as the widespread reluctance of provider organizations to share their patient care outcomes data (which would greatly enhance our ability to improve the health of individuals and populations), and the ever-present challenge of personal data security.

The pebble tossed into the pond creates rings of ripples. So it is when tossing technology into the healthcare pond. Unanticipated, even patient-endangering ripples are formed. Stated bluntly in a 2016 US Health and Human Services report, "The rapidly increasing computerization of health care has been anything but smooth, and resulted in new threats to patient safety—a cruel irony given that technological solutions have been promoted for many years as the most promising solution to medical errors."[21]

Fortunately, more and more provider organizations are awakening to these realities and adjusting their trajectories back towards success, finally understanding that technology in the absence of strategy will fail. Now recognizing that CDS solutions viewed individually rather than as integral, integrated components within a greater system will fail. Slowly appreciating that sharing data (even with competitors) is good for everyone and realizing that human (provider) behavioral obstacles to technology adoption must be addressed if reform is to succeed, the acceptance of these realities is manifest in the abandonment by many hospitals of their original CDS solutions (just as so many are now abandoning and replacing their first EHRs), followed by the strategic, selective purchase of CDS solutions which integrate, connect, and communicate across platforms, provider types, and care settings. This recent willingness of both provider organizations and HIT vendors to take a major step back to develop clear, sustainable goals, take inventory of their resources, and honestly address their challenges (both technological and human) represents a significant "second chance" for CDS solutions to successfully improve the health and healthcare of our nation.

And that's a second chance we should all encourage and support.

So what does this slow move back towards a strategic approach to CDS mean for the individual speech therapist, pharmacy technician, nurse practitioner, phlebotomist?

It means that whether you are directly involved in strategic CDS solution purchasing or implementation decisions, or if you are simply an end-user of those CDS solutions, you will be better equipped to succeed as a care provider if you understand the design of a successful CDS strategy.

The Design of a Successful Clinical Decision Support Strategy

Healthcare is enormously complex. We treat tens of millions of patients suffering from thousands of differing diseases and conditions. We prescribe from a formulary of hundreds of thousands of medications. We image with ultrasound, computed tomography (CT) scans, magnetic resonance imaging (MRI)s, fluoroscopy, angiography, nuclear scanning, positron emission tomography (PET) scans. We spend billions on laboratory systems, pathological stains, and operating room equipment. And then there are the *providers*. Hundreds of varieties of therapists and technicians and assistants and nurses and technologists and physicians and administrators. And the *technology*. So many vendors offering so many CDS solutions. Solutions for the radiology suite, the ICU, the pathology lab. For nurses. For respiratory therapists. For patients. For midwives. For use in the hospital, the office, the rehab center, the skilled nursing facility, and the home.

How are we to create sound strategies for success given all of this complexity and variability?

The same way we build houses.

I'm currently sitting at my desk in my den. As I look out the large window behind my computer monitor, I see the sun setting on the Central Florida lake that serves as my backyard. Winter here is wonderful. It's usually in the 70s with no humidity. But of course, summer is an entirely different matter. Then it's miserably hot and even more miserably humid. And it doesn't just rain in the summer. It *pours*. And the winds can get mighty strong, even hurricane strong.

Just yesterday I was feeling lucky, sitting in the plane on the Philadelphia tarmac awaiting take-off for home. An enormous northeastern storm was rapidly descending upon the region, and the airport was expected to close within hours of my departure. Sure enough, they got a ton of snow, accompanied by temperatures in the teens.

Only last week, tornados tore through parts of the Midwest. And not long ago, there was some serious flooding in the upper Northeast. And of course out on the West Coast, they recently experienced an earthquake.

The design of our houses depends significantly on where we live. It is heavily influenced by the local weather patterns (humidity, snow, heat, rain, wind) as well as by the most common regional natural threats (hurricanes, earthquakes, tornados). And so when I lived in the Midwest as a young boy, our home had a deep basement, our safe haven during terrifying tornados, and our home's walls, windows, and roof were designed to withstand the weight of the snow and to keep out the cold. My current home in Florida, on the other hand, is designed to *hold in the cold* (the air pumped out of the air conditioner vents found throughout the house). And we have those ridiculously wide rain gutters, a necessity when dealing with the enormous volume of rain that regularly dumps down during the summer. My friend in the Northeast has a bilge pump in his home's basement to automatically pump out the water that often floods his house. And for the decades I lived in California, my dwellings were literally tied to their foundations by "earthquake straps," and we had emergency gas shut-off valves and earthquake reinforcement struts.

Much like healthcare, housing architecture is complex, variable, and highly dependent on local and regional factors. Yet all of us who live in houses share some common needs: shelter from the elements, protection from Mother Nature's routine assaults. Thus, all our homes display some common design features (walls and windows and doors and roofs). And so it is with healthcare, where while modifying the design based on local needs, every provider organization requires a similar, basic architecture when building a successful CDS strategy.

By now it's clear that I love analogies. So here again, as we discuss the creation of a successful CDS strategy, I'll use one. But building a house is a bit too blasé, so let's build a *temple*. A *CDS Strategy Temple* that will stand through the years, surviving abrasive winds, pounding rain, and shifting tectonic plates.

The CDS Strategy Temple Roof: Our Strategic Vision

Our temple will need a solid roof that can endure the elements; that is, *a powerful vision* to strive for. It is obvious that the goal of our CDS Strategy is to improve the value of the care we deliver. Thus breaking "value" down into its components, our CDS Strategy vision is to achieve *high-quality, cost-efficient healthcare* (Fig. 7.5). However, we need solid, clear

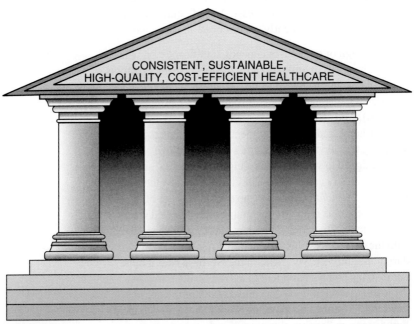

FIGURE 7.5 The roof of our Clinical Decision Support Strategy Temple, representing our strategic vision.

parameters around this goal. Such value improvement must be *consistent*, both *across care settings* (inpatient, ambulatory, home, etc.) and *across provider types*. And even consistency alone isn't enough, as *healthcare reform must be viewed as a marriage, not a wedding*. It must adjust to last and function successfully over time. That is, our CDS Strategy must drive value improvement that is *sustainable*.

Now we have a bold vision, a solid roof for our temple. And as in my earlier house building analogy, you may need to modify your institution's CDS Strategy vision to more specifically fit your local and regional provider goals. Still, I encourage you to remain bold and to take the long view when individualizing your CDS Strategy vision.

The CDS Strategy Temple Foundation: CDS Solution Requirements

No major structure can last through the ages unless it is built upon a solid foundation. Our solid CDS Strategy Temple is built upon four foundational layers. Each layer represents *a requirement which must be fulfilled for a CDS solution to be worthy of serious purchasing consideration*. And just like any foundation, all four layers (all four requirements) must be fulfilled if a CDS solution is to play a major role in your organization's value improvement strategy.

The First Foundational Layer: Evidence-Based Practice

There are several hyphenated "evidence" terms being thrown around today ("evidence-based guidelines," "evidence-informed content"). Perhaps the most comprehensive of these is "evidence-based practice." And as with any relatively new phrase, the definition and goals of "evidence-based practice" are not yet uniformly accepted. Still, to move forward in creating a successful CDS Strategy, we must utilize common terminology. I like these similar explanations of "evidence-based practice," the first more general, the second more specific to nursing, and the third a simple summation:

> "The goal of evidence-based practice (EBP) is the integration of: (a) clinical expertise/expert opinion, (b) external scientific evidence, and (c) client/patient/caregiver values to provide high-quality services reflecting the interests, values, needs, and choices of the individuals we serve."[22]

⊙ PEARL

CDS solutions come in many varieties and formats. However, the most successful CDS strategies start with a bold, powerful vision including *the consistent delivery of sustainable, high quality, cost efficient healthcare.*

"An ongoing process by which evidence, nursing theory, and the practitioners' clinical expertise are critically evaluated and considered, in conjunction with patient involvement, to provide delivery of optimum nursing care for the individual."[23]

"EBP is the integration of clinical expertise, patient values, and the best research evidence into the decision-making process for patient care."[24]

Thus whether you are a speech therapist, pharmacist, occupational or physical therapist, nutritionist, other allied health professional, or nurse, patient care today must be founded upon an evidence-based practice approach. That is, the evaluation, treatment, and overall medical care provided our patients must be grounded in scientific evidence supported by clinical expertise and influenced by patient input. The best such scientific evidence and clinical expertise is *current,* offered by *credible* sources, and based on *scientifically rigorous* clinical trials. The pinnacle of such scientific evidence is the prospective, double-blinded, randomized, controlled clinical trial of adequate statistical sample size. The reality is that such solidly designed clinical trials have not been performed to evaluate "the best care approach" for the majority of clinical conditions, and we're often left to sort through less-well designed clinical trials and simple published case reports. Still, especially when vetted through a valid peer-review process (and subsequently published or presented), such "evidence" is often quite useful. And again, evidence-based practice suggests that even the most impressive scientific evidence should be tempered by our own professional experience. Of course, this is where we are at risk of entering a quagmire: when does our professional care provider experience trump the scientific evidence published in a peer-reviewed journal article or presented as a professional society guideline? Each of us must seek our own answer to this question when it arises, but it is worth recognizing that the results from well-designed studies of large patient populations is powerful, even if those results differ from our own limited experience. Finally, we must add to the evidence-based information and our professional experience the patient's own values and needs.

So in the end, "evidence-based practice" isn't quite as simple or objective as it sounds.

Still, the requirement that CDS solutions incorporate or support current, credible, evidence-based practice is

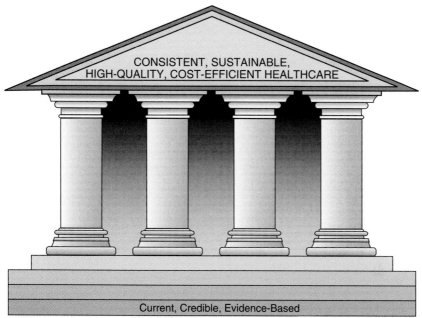

FIGURE 7.6 The first Foundational Layer of our Clinical Decision Support Strategy Temple.

foundational to a healthy and sustainable CDS Strategy (Fig. 7.6), and you should be skeptical of the value offered by any CDS solution that does not utilize a rigorous, evidence grading system or that does not regularly update its content.

The Second Foundational Layer: Serving All Major Providers

While newer CDS solutions such as care plans and clinical pathways seek to better support interprofessional care delivery, most of today's CDS solutions are still provider-type specific. Not only are these tools aimed at a narrow audience (pharmacists, physical therapists, nurse educators, etc.), they often fail to appreciate (let alone incorporate) interprofessional care concepts or functionalities. Still, as we move towards the greater availability of truly interprofessional CDS solutions, we must also remember that today's "best patient care" requires CDS solutions supporting all major provider types, not just physicians (Fig. 7.7). Thus we have the second foundational layer on which our robust CDS Strategy Temple is built. (We will discuss these major provider types more specifically in the next section, *The Four Pillars*.)

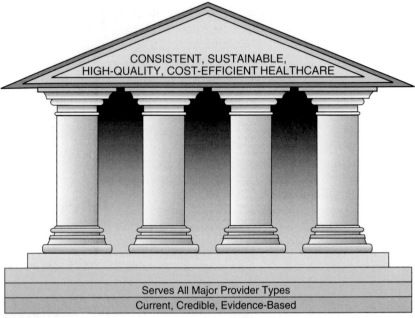

FIGURE 7.7 The second Foundational Layer of our Clinical Decision Support Strategy Temple.

The Third Foundational Layer: Availability at All Points of Patient Care

Healthcare is no longer confined to the hospital and doctor's office. Just take a quick look through the lay press:

> "With 7,800 retail stores and a presence in almost every state, CVS Health has [become] the country's biggest operator of health clinics . . ."[25]
> *The Seattle Times,* August 2015

> "Top 10 Healthcare Companies in the U.S. Based on Revenue:
> #7. Walgreens Boots Alliance ($76.4 billion)
> #1. CVS Health ($139.4 billion)."[26]
> *Global Healthcare,* 2015

Healthcare is moving at lightning speed from the physician's world into the retail world. From the traditional provider's workflow into the consumer living flow. Even into places of patient employment (with support of both employers and governmental agencies).[27] And into the patient home (including care activities traditionally

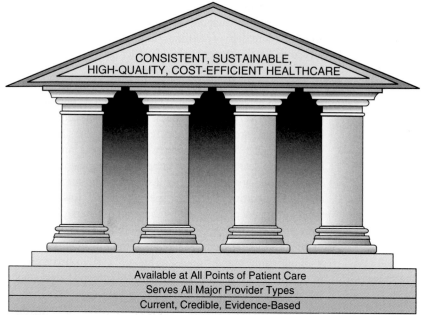

FIGURE 7.8 The third Foundational Layer of our Clinical Decision Support Strategy Temple.

confined to the hospital or medical office setting, such as IV drug administration).[28]

And healthcare reform is aggressively shifting the balance away from the traditional inpatient to the outpatient care setting, as physical therapy, chemotherapy infusion, surgery, urgent care, advanced imaging, and hundreds of other formerly in-hospital care activities are now offered in ambulatory provider venues.

In this new world, healthcare must move seamlessly between provider types (the second Foundational Layer) across all care settings. This third Foundational Layer thus demands that to be of greatest value, CDS solutions must empower providers in driving toward our goal of consistent, sustainable high-quality, cost efficient healthcare *wherever that care is being delivered to our patients* (Fig. 7.8).

The Fourth Foundational Layer: Minimally Disruptive to Provider Workflow

I was serving as an executive in a large healthcare system when we began replacing the many EHRs used by the various providers whose small practices we had acquired. Our intent was good: to place every one of our dozens of ambulatory care practices onto the same EHR platform as used in our many hospitals to improve patient care across all of our care delivery settings. One of our busiest practices served pediatric surgical spine disorder patients. In addition to the surgeon, the practice included a physician assistant, a physical therapist, an occupational therapist, a pediatric social worker, two nurses, two coders, and a receptionist (theirs was a very busy practice). Before being acquired by our healthcare network, this team of providers had for years utilized a "cottage industry" EHR; that is, an EHR specifically designed for use in pediatric surgical practices. For the allied health professionals, nurses, the surgeon, and administrative staff, that "specialty EHR" was exactly what they needed, designed by those who understood the workflow in a busy pediatric surgical practice. Several months following the replacement of their original EHR with our name-brand, "one-size-fits-all" system (from one of the largest EHR vendors in the world), the pediatric spine surgery team shared with us data they had collected which demonstrated *the significant loss in productivity that their practice had suffered* since the technological change. The therapists, nurses, physician assistant, coders, surgeon . . . all identified that the significant extra time needed to navigate their new "one-size-fits-all" EHR was the source of their dramatically decreased office productivity (and associated projected *$100,000 reduction in annual practice revenue).* Needless to say, the practice team was not pleased.

In fact, this interprofessional subspecialty care team's claims are consistent with published reports demonstrating the negative correlation between EHR use and practice productivity. One study primarily supported by the American Medical Association focusing on physician productivity found that "During the office day, physicians spent 27.0% of their total time on direct clinical face time with patients and 49.2% of their time on EHR and desk work."[29] And as the pediatric spine surgery team exemplified, EHR technology can be problematic not only for doctors, but also for nurses[30] and allied health professionals. In fact, some EHR systems have developed such a bad reputation that their use impacts hospital staffing: according to a 2014 *Healthcare IT News* report,[31] "A poorly implemented EHR with chaotic processes and bungling IT support is becoming a detriment to hospital nurse retention and recruitment."

And EHRs were just the first of the new healthcare reform technologies to generate significant frustration (even anger) among providers. As more and more CDS solutions continue to be piled on top of the EHR, many allied health professionals, nurses, and physicians are feeling that even more patient face-to-face time is being stolen. Patients often feel the same: my elderly aunt told me that virtually her entire recent cardiology office visit involved staring at her providers' backs, as first the nurse, then the medical assistant, and finally the cardiologist each spent most of her office visit time facing the computer while asking her questions.

In the end, many providers and patients feel that today's healthcare technology has taken away from the provider-patient relationship, from the human-to-human interaction that lies at the heart of healthcare. Thus it is easy to see why many of us roll our eyes when our hospitals introduce us to yet another CDS solution that we are required to use to "improve patient care."

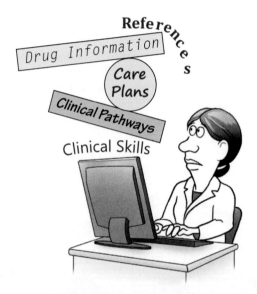

Still, we must look past real or perceived reduced individual provider (or provider team) efficiency. We must see the forest and not just the trees. We must truly understand the potential that CDS solutions offer to dramatically improve our healthcare system. Even now, studies have begun to demonstrate not only the benefits of EHR adoption,[32,33,34] but improvements in patient care outcomes associated with use of CDS solutions.[35] Perhaps the apparently binary effects of healthcare IT (EHRs and CDS solutions) is best summarized in a 2015 report published by the *Agency for Healthcare Research and Quality* (AHRQ, a part of the US Department of Health and Human Services): "Although significant obstacles prevent many primary care practices from using health IT for QI [quality improvement], practices in diverse settings have demonstrated it is possible and pays off in improved processes of care and patient outcomes."[36]

It is too much to ask that today's CDS solutions improve provider workflow, productivity, and efficiency. Truth be told, most of us would be happy if the new technologies just *didn't slow us down.* But for now, we need to accept that *while CDS solutions may reduce direct patient-face time and our productivity, the promise offered by such systems in terms of improved patient safety, consistently better patient outcomes, and cost savings, is enormous and well worth the frustration and challenges we are currently experiencing today, early in the CDS age.*

That being said, there remains significant variability into the provider workflow disruption associated with differing CDS solutions. So while we await future solutions which more seamlessly integrate within the provider workflow, today's technology realities form the basis of the fourth and final Foundational Layer of our CDS Strategy Temple: the most powerful CDS solutions are those that providers more readily adopt into their daily care activities, and those are the CDS solutions that are *minimally disruptive to provider workflow* (Fig. 7.9).

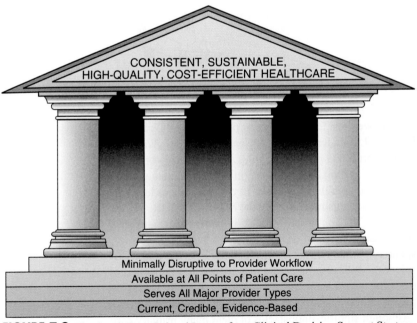

CONSISTENT, SUSTAINABLE, HIGH-QUALITY, COST-EFFICIENT HEALTHCARE

Minimally Disruptive to Provider Workflow
Available at All Points of Patient Care
Serves All Major Provider Types
Current, Credible, Evidence-Based

FIGURE 7.9 The fourth Foundational Layer of our Clinical Decision Support Strategy Temple.

For now, we need to accept that while CDS solutions may reduce direct patient-face time and our productivity, the promise offered by such systems in terms of improved patient safety, consistently better patient outcomes, and cost savings, is enormous and well worth the frustration and challenges we are currently experiencing today, early in the CDS age.

Thus I encourage you to seek out opportunities to participate in your hospital's prepurchase evaluation of CDS solutions that you will be asked to incorporate into your daily care workflow. Go and see for yourself in action in the real world any solution under consideration (vendor demonstrations, by their very nature, always show the solution in a favorable light); that is, require that the vendor arrange for you to see their CDS solution in use in a healthcare setting similar to yours. Shadow your provider counterpart and evaluate the impact of the CDS solution on his or her care activities. Remember, CDS solutions often do slow us down (that's just the current reality); the important question is: is the disruption in provider workflow caused by the CDS solution *minimal enough for now to make the patient care benefit worthwhile?*

The Four Pillars: The Providers

The second Foundational Layer demands that to be of greatest value, CDS solutions must "serve all major provider types." As discussed in the opening chapters of this book, the definition and responsibilities of "Provider" have changed significantly with the healthcare reform movement, expanding the "Provider" list dramatically. It is the "major provider types" that are represented in our model by Four Pillars. Supporting the roof of our CDS Strategy Temple above (our CDS vision) and planted firmly on top of our four Foundational Layers below (requirements of our CDS solutions), the Four Pillars each represent a "major provider" group that must be empowered through CDS solutions if we are to fulfill our CDS Strategy vision.

Actually, there are *five* pillars…

That fifth pillar is "Physicians." Obviously physicians, the traditional (and in the past, the sole) "Provider," must be empowered by CDS solutions if we are to achieve our strategic goals. But *as this book is a guide for nurses and allied health professionals, in this CDS Strategy Temple model, the "Physician" pillar will not be pictured.*

Of course, the most complete and likely most impactful CDS solutions would be designed to include each and every type of allied health professional and nurse. But that is not how CDS solution vendors have created their products (as market size considerations are driving forces in solution development). And for my purposes, I will narrow the "major provider" list even further, ingloriously lumping several individual provider types into single pillar. So with apologies, but for the sake of understanding, here are the Four Pillars:

The First Pillar: Nurses

Without a doubt, *nurses are now playing an increasingly critical role in improving the quality and cost efficiency of patient care.*[37] It is thus absolutely necessary that CDS solutions are designed based on the unique ways in which nurses understand, analyze, adopt, and incorporate evidence-based information and care guidelines into their practice. Just pick up a credible nursing journal and compare the way articles are written and data presented against an article from a major physician journal. Nurses have their own specific and complex care workflows that integrate direct patient care activities, care transitions, regulated work shifts, indirect patient care activities, and significant support of other provider activities and schedules. As a result, nurses have unique needs within an integrated CDS system, demanding dedicated CDS solutions and/or nursing-centric portions of broader, interprofessional CDS solutions (such as care plans and clinical pathways). And again, all such nurse-empowering CDS solutions must seek to achieve the common CDS Strategy vision (our Temple roof) while meeting the requirements of our four Foundational Layers.

The Second Pillar: Pharmacy Health Professionals

The reduction (in fact, elimination) of preventable medical errors linked to medication mistakes[38,39] is one of the major goals of healthcare reform. The sheer volume of ordered inpatient and ambulatory medications, combined with the significant knowledge required to safely evaluate and then dispense both pharmaceuticals, not to mention the rapidly expanding medication formulary, demands that "Pharmacy Health Professionals" be represented by one of the Four Pillars within our CDS Strategy Temple. Add to the complex and numerous challenges currently facing pharmacy health professionals the expansion of medication delivery sites to include retail centers, places of work, and the patient home, and it becomes clear that this group of healthcare professionals (like nurses) require dedicated CDS solutions (or, again, focused portions of interprofessional CDS solutions) if we are to maximize the value of healthcare delivery.

The Third Pillar: Allied Health Professionals

Yes, this third pillar can easily be separated into dozens of pillars, as there are so many types of specialized allied health professional working across the expanding care settings and who are critical to successful healthcare reform. Still, rather than offer CDS solutions specific to physical therapists, dieticians, speech therapists, ultrasonographers, and the many more types of allied health professionals, vendors now include various allied health professionals into the broader, interprofessional CDS solutions (such as care plans and clinical pathways). What is necessary to achieve successful healthcare reform are CDS solutions that empower all allied health professionals across the care continuum. Only when a CDS strategy includes physical therapists, radiographers, speech therapist, dieticians, sonographers, and the dozens of other allied health professionals will we realize consistent, sustainable, high quality, cost efficient healthcare.

PEARL

Major provider groups include nurses, pharmacy health professionals (including pharmacist), allied health professionals, and patients (as well as physicians).

The Fourth Pillar: Patients

If we are truly to not only improve the value of our healthcare, but better our nation's *health,* "Patients" must be given and must accept the responsibility as the "Ultimate Provider." There is only so much that an occupational therapist or physician assistant can do to improve any patient's health in the few minutes spent[40] in direct contact with that patient. Patients themselves, supported by their loved ones and their provider partners, must take ownership of their health. To do so, patients (like all provider types) must be supported by easily accessible, highly intuitive CDS solutions. From the simplest "Symptom Checker" or "Appointment Scheduler" to the most complex, patient-specific "Risk Calculator" or "Health Planner," today's patients already have access to numerous CDS solutions. What is often lacking is integration of these solutions within the CDS Strategy used by the patient's medical providers across the patient's care delivery settings. In moving forward, we must aggressively include CDS solutions for our patients into our overall CDS Strategy Temple.

The Complete CDS Strategy Temple

So there it is: our *CDS Strategy Temple* (Fig. 7.10). A basic design to guide your organization's CDS solution purchasing decisions (in which I encourage you to volunteer and participate!) and a primer for the use of these solutions in your practice. But there is still one more aspect of a CDS Strategy that you must understand: *seatbelts and airbags*.

The Pull and Push of CDS Solutions

It is illegal to manufacture a car for sale in the United States that does not include functional seatbelts for the driver and all passengers. As of 2017, there are seatbelt laws in 49 of the 50 states requiring that the driver buckle up whenever operating the vehicle (and in 28 states, requiring that all passengers buckle as well)[41]. And yet according to the National Highway Traffic Safety Administration,[42] 49% of the over 21,000 killed in car accidents in 2014 were known to not be wearing their seatbelts at the time of their deaths. Why did they die? Because, like 13% of all Americans, these 10,000-plus individuals *failed to buckle up.*

Seatbelts are what I call *pull solutions.* That is, *seatbelts require active participation by the target user if the desired benefit is to be realized.* Buckle up, and your chance of surviving a car crash rises dramatically, and the significance of any crash-related injury drops precipitously. Don't buckle up? Your car may as well be seatbelt-less.

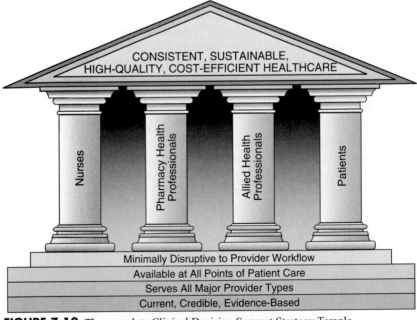

FIGURE 7.10 The complete Clinical Decision Support Strategy Temple.

Many CDS solutions are pull solutions. They require the user (allied health professional, nurse, physician, patient) to *actively seek answers* to patient care questions. This is often not only challenging, but it can be dangerous, because in this world of rapidly expanding patient care information, we *providers often don't know what we don't know.*

My mother called from the hospital, her voice frantic. This was surprising, given that she had entered the hospital that morning as long planned in preparation for elective spine surgery the following morning.

"What's wrong?" I asked, only minimally concerned, as there was no reason to believe my mother, electively hospitalized in a renowned academic medical center, was in any real danger.

"I keep having dry heaves," she said, clearly frightened. "And I've been nauseous for hours. And my belly hurts."

My own personal bias (that of a physician, meaning I often feel less-than-appropriate concern over symptoms in loved ones than I feel for strangers in the emergency room) began to lessen upon hearing these very specific physical complaints.

"What did the nurse say?" I asked.

"She said it's nothing . . . just presurgery nerves."

"That doesn't make sense," I replied. My mother obviously agreed, hence her call to me. She had undergone countless orthopedic operations during her adult life, a result of her rheumatoid arthritis.

"Did you get something for your nausea?" I asked.

"Yes, just a few minutes ago," Mom answered.

"Do you want me to speak with your nurse?"

"No . . . not yet," she said, seeming to calm a bit. "I'll call you back if I'm not feeling better soon."

Ninety minutes later, my mother called again.

"I'm still nauseous, and my belly still hurts a bit," she explained. "Now my nurse says it's my gallbladder, and that she'll tell the general surgery team in the morning."

Now, I had by then cared for dozens and dozens and dozens of patients suffering from acute and chronic inflammation of their gallbladders as a result of gallstones. And I knew that (A) this wasn't gallbladder disease and (B) something potentially serious was going on with my mom. And so I told my mother that I would call the nurses' station, speak with her nurse, and call her back in a few minutes.

"What's your assessment of my mother's ongoing nausea and mild abdominal pain?" I asked her primary nurse 2 minutes later.

"Gallstones," she replied confidently.

"I'm concerned it's something else, something else acute. Something much more dangerous."

"What is that?" she asked, sounding unconvinced.

"I think she is having a heart attack."

Momentary silence, followed by "I don't think so, Dr. Edelstein. I know she's your mother, so it's not surprising that you're overly concerned about her symptoms."

Mind you she was not condescending when she said this to me. She was truly trying to calm me and continue caring for her patient.

"In my experience, your mother's symptoms are consistent with gallstones, not with a myocardial infarction [heart attack]."

To make a long story short, she was a competent, experienced floor nurse. But of the several possible medical explanations for my mother's now hours-long nausea, dry heaves, and abdominal pain, this nurse had allowed her personal experience and limited clinical knowledge to bias to her conclusion. She had not for a moment considered accessing the hospital's on-line reference solution to identify other possible clinical explanations for my mother's symptoms. Had she done so, had this dedicated, well-trained nurse recognized that she might not know what was going on with my mother and chosen to utilize the available CDS, she would likely have rapidly determined that my mother's symptoms were, in fact, *classic for women suffering acute cardiac ischemia.*

Unfortunately, my mother's nurse didn't know what she didn't know. Thus she was entirely unaware that my mother was not suffering from her first acute gallstone attack. She was having a myocardial infarction.

Fortunately, after hours of this classic presentation of cardiac ischemia in a woman, I convinced the nurse (a mild term for how I actually acted) to call the cardiac fellow who, while the EKG rolled across the computer screen, ordered her team to prepare for an emergency catheterization of my mother's coronary vessels.

Fortunately, my mother survived her very real heart attack.

And she's never had a problem with her gallbladder.

The nurse who cared for my mother is a good care provider. And she truly believed that she understood exactly what was going on with her patient. But her own bias quietly crept in, preventing her from accepting that there was another explanation for my mother's symptoms, an etiology of which she was unaware. Patients are injured every day, and large sums of money are wasted, because nurses, pharmacists, therapists, physicians, and other allied health professionals never bother to search for current, credible information simply because *they don't know that they don't know* the best thing to do when caring for their patients. Hundreds of thousands of preventable deaths annually, and tens of thousands of avoidable complications each and every day, are the result of provider ignorance not only in appropriate care delivery, but *ignorance in not recognizing that they don't know what is the current "best care" for their patients.*

This is the very real danger of relying solely on CDS pull solutions: they require that the provider recognizes his or her lack of patient care knowledge and, therefore, actively seeks access to current, credible, patient care information. The nurse practitioner who knows nothing of inflammatory breast cancer will not search a CDS pull solution for "tender, red skin over the breast in young women" when evaluating a young woman with tender, erythematous (red) skin over a portion of her breast. More likely (and I have personally seen this), the patient will be incorrectly diagnosed with and treated for a superficial skin infection, delaying the treatment of her actual aggressive, rapidly progressive malignancy. The physician assistant who fails to consider that patients can simultaneously harbor both mildly bleeding hemorrhoids and a mildly bleeding rectal cancer won't likely look up "evaluating bright red blood per rectum" on a CDS pull solution when seeing friable (easily bleeding) internal hemorrhoids on examination of a 54-year-old, delaying the diagnosis and treatment of the rectal cancer (this I have seen many times as well).

This is the very real danger of relying solely on CDS pull solutions: they require that the provider recognizes his or her lack of patient care knowledge and, therefore, actively seeks access to current, credible, patient care information.

Even when a provider recognizes a knowledge gap and voluntarily searches for information, if that information is either not current and/or not from a credible source, the results can be disastrous. A common example is when providers search on noncredible sources such as Wikipedia (demonstrated to offer inappropriate patient care information)[4] and similar websites. Even more dramatic is when patients "site shop," seeking the answer they desire rather than the most credible care guidance.

The call from the emergency room to see a patient "with a large cancer" was nothing unusual. What did surprise me is how the ER nurse described the patient.

"He smells awful," she said. "In fact, that's why he's here."

"You mean, he wants to know why he smells?" I asked.

"No," she replied in a whispered tone. *"He was asked to get off of the airplane because so many people were complaining about his stench."*

She wasn't exaggerating. Mr. Richards was flying to Dallas and had a stopover in San Diego. At that time, the cabin crew had told him (as kindly as they could) that he would have to deplane, as his odor was too much for the other passengers to take. They suggested (and he complied) that he immediately seek medical attention.

I had practiced surgery long enough to recognize the smell before even opening the curtains which separated my new patient from the busy ER. It was the unique, overwhelming odor of dead tissue exposed to the air.

Mr. Richards was a pleasant, intelligent, soft-spoken accountant who appeared embarrassed to be bothering anyone with his medical concerns. Upon initial inspection, it was obvious to me that he was suffering from a very advanced malignancy: he was overly (dangerously) thin, typical of advanced cancer patients. Seeing him standing uncomfortably against the exam table (rather than sitting on it) told me even more. These immediate images, combined with the pungent odor from exposed, dying tissue, led to my first postintroductory question.

"How long have you had your rectal cancer?"

Mr. Richards was silent for a moment, assessing my perhaps-surprising initial inquiry.

"A little over a year," he answered.

And so Mr. Richards' story unfolded. He had experienced some minor rectal bleeding about 14 months earlier. As he was in his 50s, his astute primary care physician scheduled a colonoscopy, which revealed a rectal cancer. Referred to cancer specialists in his community, Mr. Richards had listened attentively and accepted the recommendation for preoperative radiation and chemotherapy and postoperative chemotherapy based on his cancer stage. The proposed surgery, however, was a different matter.

Given how distal (close to the anal opening) his malignancy was growing, the surgeon could not guarantee that after surgery Mr. Richards wouldn't be left with a colostomy (in which an end of large intestine is brought through the abdominal wall, allowing stool to flow into a pouch attached by adhesive to the skin of the abdomen; this is necessary when removing a cancer includes removing the anal musculature, meaning that the patient can no longer empty their bowel through the anus). Despite understanding that a colostomy was far from a certainty, Mr. Richards just could not accept it.

Thus began Mr. Richards' journey with free, online "cancer care" pull solutions. He searched nonstop to find alternatives to the recommended surgery in an attempt to cure him. I emphasize "cure," because *Mr. Richards absolutely wanted to be cured.* But equally, he wanted to avoid even the smallest risk that he would awaken from surgery to a life with a colostomy bag collecting his stool in a pouch stuck to his stomach. And so he searched under terms such as, "rectal cancer cure without surgery" and "curing rectal cancer without colostomy," pulling information from the worldwide web that allowed him to piece together an acceptable plan: curing his rectal cancer without any possibility of his needing a colostomy.

And it is within Mr. Richards' journey that we so clearly see the dangers of freely available, online "healthcare" pull solutions. He found a "doctor" who offered a "cure" without any surgery at all. In fact, even without any radiation or chemotherapy. And so Mr. Richards had been shelling out heaps of cash to this provider. All without spending a single moment under a radiation machine, in an operating room, or in a chemotherapy bay.

And his rectal cancer, likely curable when first diagnosed 14 months earlier, had grown into a massive tumor that now protruded out through his anus, the overlying malignant tissue dying in the room air and generating the horrific smell, the growth preventing him from sitting. And now his cancer had spread, first to the lymph nodes adjacent to his large bowel and eventually to his liver.

And so Mr. Richards died not long after we first met in the ER. He died because of several factors. First of all, the pull solutions Mr. Richards eventually followed to guide his cancer care were from *noncredible sources.* Second (and related to the first), Mr. Richards' *own bias guided which pull solutions he chose to believe in.* That is, he went into his pull solution search already having determined that he needed to be cured, but that any surgical treatment could not include any risk of a colostomy.

His treatment? Drinking wheat grass juice supplemented by other, nonspecified "anticancer nutrients" several times each day while undergoing multiple "blood tests" performed by his "doctor" several times each month.

The exotic location where Mr. Richards received his alternative (and eventually fatal) care?

Cleveland.

Patients, nurses, allied health professionals, physicians . . . we are all human. Subject to internal biases most favorable to our own training and experiences and expectations. As such, we must be aware of these potential hazards when utilizing CDS pull solutions to answer our patient care questions.

Thus whether a traditional provider or a patient, CDS pull solutions have many potential pitfalls: the provider may fail to recognize what they don't know and, therefore, never seek to fill their knowledge gap; the provider may seek information from sources which are either noncredible and/or do not offer current, evidence-based information; the provider's own bias may lead him or her to ignore current, credible, evidence-based guidance, seeking "credible" information consistent with that conscious or subconscious bias.

Still, when lumped together, the great danger posed to our patients by CDS pull solutions is this: *we don't know what we don't know.* And yet when correctly accessed and utilized, CDS pull solutions absolutely can and do improve the quality and cost efficiency of healthcare delivery. So how do we maximize the significant value of CDS pull solutions, given these real challenges?

We return to our car analogy.

Fortunately, our cars don't just have seatbelts. They have *airbags.* Driver airbags. Passenger airbags. Front airbags. Side airbags. You start your car, the airbags arm. You hit the car ahead of you (or a tree, or a cow), and the airbags deploy. No activation button. Nothing. *Automatic.* Safety that is *pushed* to you and your passengers. And, fortunately, there are *CDS push solutions.*

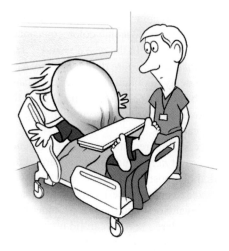

CDS push solutions are incredibly powerful, automatically pushing current, credible, evidence-based care information directly to the provider at the point of care. Order Sets, Care Plans, and Clinical Pathways exemplify currently available, powerful CDS push solutions. CDS push solutions recommend actions that the provider should consider (whether or not the provider is aware of such recommendations).

When initiating a Care Plan for a young woman with a tender, red breast, the nurse practitioner would automatically be presented with queries and recommendations based on current, credible, evidence-based guidelines[43]:

- Does the affected tissue cover a third or more of the breast?
- What is the patient's ethnicity?
- Does the affected skin appear to have ridges or pits?
- Is the nipple inverted?
- Are there swollen lymph nodes under the adjacent arm or adjacent collarbone?

The nurse practitioner who knows little or nothing of inflammatory breast cancer (and who doesn't know what she doesn't know) would likely never have considered (let alone actively searched for) such clinical information. But *pushed* to the nurse practitioner, this CDS guidance empowers the nurse practitioner to rapidly reach the correct diagnosis, allowing immediate treatment planning for this aggressive malignancy.

A Clinical Pathway for minor lower gastrointestinal bleeding that actively *pushes CDS guidance* will remind the physician assistant to perform a digital rectal exam on the 54-year-old patient *even in the presence of visibly bleeding hemorrhoids* and recommend to the physician assistant that the patient undergo endoscopic colorectal cancer screening (unless performed within the past 5 years).[44] The Clinical Pathway *pushes appropriate diagnostic recommendations,* preventing a delay in diagnosis of the rectal cancer.

CDS push solutions also recommend what the evidence suggests providers should not do in their diagnostic and therapeutic care.

An Order Set that recommends the emergency room medical assistant *not* include bilateral carotid ultrasound in the initial diagnostic work-up of a patient with a history of generalized syncope benefits the patient (saving time to appropriate evaluation and treatment), other patients (who are in line to undergo needed carotid ultrasound), and the system (reducing unnecessary costs of care).

In addition to "don't do care activities," the Order Set will guide the medical assistant in ordering appropriate initial diagnostic tests,[45] such as an EKG and, potentially, a Holter monitor study.

So CDS push solutions inform and guide providers to providing the best patient care, including avoiding unnecessary diagnostic and/or therapeutic care activities that are of no value.

And just as drivers and passengers are safest when traveling in cars with their seatbelts buckled and airbags functioning, *the most powerful CDS strategy includes both pull and push solutions.* In fact, *CDS pull and push solutions function together.* When suddenly made aware by a CDS *push* solution of a recommended diagnostic test, therapeutic procedure, or of a medical condition, patient risk, disease, or condition previously unknown or not considered, the provider can then (or at a later time) seek additional information and knowledge by actively exploring the topic using a CDS *pull* solution. This is evident in the example from earlier in this chapter:

A general surgeon plans to perform a partial colon resection on a 57-year-old man diagnosed with a cancer of the right colon. Fortunately, his CDS push solution (an Order Set for colon cancer patients admitted for surgery) recommends that this patient first undergo a blood test to potentially diagnose a genetic syndrome more common in younger colon cancer patients with right-sided malignancies. The patient's blood test confirms that he suffers from the syndrome.

The surgeon now accesses a CDS pull solution (a Reference Solution) and learns that the procedure he originally recommended is not the appropriate operation, as it places the patient at a high risk of a second colon cancer in the future. He educates himself and subsequently performs the recommended surgical procedure, to the benefit of his patient.

CDS push solutions are often dependent on CDS pull solutions, as the latter are frequently the source of the evidence-based guidelines incorporated into the former (i.e., those who create push solutions such as Order Sets, Care Plans, and Clinical Pathways create the pushed guidance based on information retrieved from CDS pull solutions).

While far from complete (especially because the availability and capabilities of CDS solutions continue to rapidly expand), here are some examples of CDS pull and push solutions set within the framework of our CDS Strategy Temple, for Nurses (Fig. 7.11), Pharmacy Health Professionals (Fig. 7.12), Allied Health Professionals (Fig. 7.13), and Patients (Fig. 7.14).

PEARL

Patients, providers, and healthcare organizations are best served by a combination of CDS pull solutions (which require the user to actively search for information) and CDS push solutions (which automatically push patient and scenario-specific information to the provider).

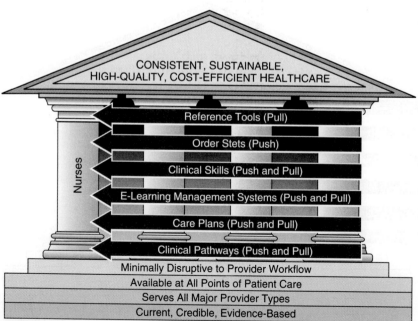

FIGURE 7.11 Examples of Clinical Decision Support pull and push solutions for Nurses.

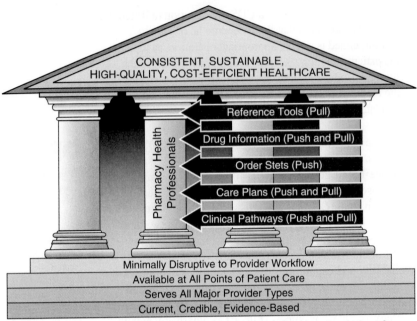

FIGURE 7.12 Examples of Clinical Decision Support pull and push solutions for Pharmacy Health Professionals (including pharmacists).

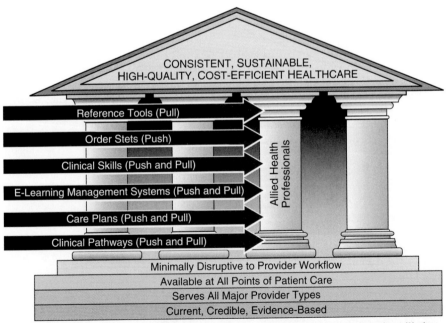

FIGURE 7.13 Examples of Clinical Decision Support pull and push solutions for Allied Health Professionals.

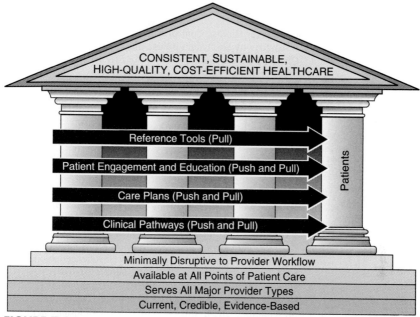

FIGURE 7.14 Examples of Clinical Decision Support pull and push solutions for the "Ultimate Provider": Patients.

CDS Solutions: Putting It All Together

While this chapter may seem to you a bit long for a "guide," the reality is that we have only just scratched the tip of the iceberg that is CDS. And whether you are a healthcare student, a new provider, or an experienced care practitioner, CDS solutions are now universally present tools in our care delivery world and, more and more, integral parts of our provider workflow.

While it can be challenging, even frustrating and angering, to be asked (or required) to master and incorporate CDS solutions into your everyday practice, and while it is true that, at least initially, the use of such technological systems often actually reduces your productivity and worsens your efficiency, remember the ultimate goal here: *consistent, sustainable, high-quality, cost-efficient healthcare for our patients.*

In other words, every once in a while (and particularly when you're frustrated), return and visit the roof (the strategic vision) of your organization's CDS Strategy Temple.

References

1. Centers for Disease Control and Prevention. (online); https://www.cdc.gov/ehrmeaningfuluse/introduction.html.
2. Charles D, King J, et al. *Adoption of Electronic Health Record Systems Among U.S. Non-federal Acute Care Hospitals: 2008-2012*; March, 2013. ONC Data Brief No. 9.
3. Hayes TO. Are Electronic Health Records Worth the Cost of Implementation? American Action Forum (online) https://www.americanactionforum.org/research/are-electronic-medical-records-worth-the-costs-of-implementation/.
4. Hasty RT, Garbalosa RC, Barbato VA, et al. Wikipedia vs peer-reviewed medical literature for information about the 10 most costly medical conditions. *J Am Osteopath Assoc.* 2014;114:368–373.
5. Ware M, Mabe M. *The STM Report: An Overview of Scientific and Scholarly Journal Publishing*. STM (online); 2015. http://www.stm-assoc.org/2015_02_20_STM_Report_2015.pdf.
6. Boon S. *21st Century Science Overload*. Canadian Science Publishing (online); 2016. http://www.cdnsciencepub.com/blog/21st-century-science-overload.aspx.
7. Hart K. *Medicare Documentation for the Rehabilitation Patient*. Harmony Healthcare International, Inc. (online presentation); 2014. Slide 47. https://www.slideshare.net/HarmonyHealthcareInternational/medicare-documentation-for-the-rehabilitation-patient-evidence-of-progress.
8. Sokol DK, Hettige S. Poor handwriting remains a significant problem in medicine. *J R Soc Med.* 2006;99:645–646.
9. Patel NR. Clinical Informatics. In: Hazinski MF, ed. *Nursing Care of the Critically Ill Child.* 3rd ed.Philadelphia: Mosby; 2013.
10. Abramson EL, Kaushal R. Computerized provider order entry and patient safety. *Pediatr Clin North Am.* 2012;59:1247–1255.
11. U.S. Department of Health and Human Services: Agency for Healthcare Research and Quality (online) 2015; https://psnet.ahrq.gov/primers/primer/23/medication-errors.
12. Wachter RM. Quality of Care and Patient Safety. *Goldman-Cecil Medicine.* 25th ed. Philadelphia: Saunders; 2016.
13. Guise JM, Segel S. Teamwork in Obstetric Critical Care. *Best Pract Res Clin Obstet Gynaecol.* 2008;22:937–951.
14. Pettker C, Funai E. Patient safety in obstetrics. *Creasy & Resnik's Maternal-Fetal Medicine.* 7th ed. Philadelphia: Saunders; 2014.
15. Stanford University (online) http://online.stanford.edu/course/machine-learning.
16. Winter AF, Ammenwerth E, Bott OJ, et al. Strategic information management plans: the basis for systematic information management in hospitals. *Inter J Med Informatics.* 2001;64:99–109.
17. Bush M, Lederer AL, Li X, Palmisano J, Rao S. The alignment of information systems with organizational objectives and strategies in health care. *Inter J Med Informatics.* 2009;78:446–456.
18. Jenkins MK. *Why Do Healthcare IT Projects Fail?* Physicians Practice (online); 2011. http://www.physicianspractice.com/blog/why-do-healthcare-it-projects-fail.

19. U.S. Department of Health and Human Services, Agency for Healthcare Research and Quality, 2016 (online) https://psnet. ahrq.gov/primers/primer/28/alert-fatigue.

20. Wadhwa R, Fridsma DB, Saul MI, et al. Analysis of a failed clinical decision support system for management of congestive heart failure. *AMIA Annu Symp Proc.* 2008;6:773–777.

21. U.S. Department of Health and Human Services, Agency for Healthcare Research and Quality, 2016 (online) https://psnet. ahrq.gov/primers/primer/28/alert-fatigue.

22. Sackett D, et al. Evidence-Based Medicine. In: *How to Practice and Teach EBM.* 2nd ed.Edinburgh: Churchill Livingstone; 2000:1.

23. Scott K, McSherry R. Evidence based nursing: clarifying the concepts for nurses in practice. *J Clin Nurs.* 2009;18:1085–1095.

24. University of North Carolina Health Sciences Library (online) http://hsl.lib.unc.edu/services/ evidence-based-practice-resources.

25. The Seattle Times, August 2015.

26. Global Healthcare, 2015 (online) http:// www.healthcareglobal.com/top10/2110/ Top-10-healthcare-companies-in-the-US-based-on-revenue.

27. Centers for Disease Control and Prevention. (online) https:// www.cdc.gov/workplacehealthpromotion/index.html.

28. Health IT News, 2016 (online) http:// www.continuumofcarenews.com/blog/ hospitals-moving-care-delivery-patient-homes.

29. Sinsky C, Colligan L, Li L, et al. Allocation of physician time in ambulatory practice: a time and motion study in 4 specialties. *Ann Intern Med.* 2016;165:753–760.

30. Nelson R. AJN reports: electronic health records: useful tools or high-tech headache? *Am J Nurs.* 2007;107:25–26.

31. Health IT News, 2014 (online) http://www.healthcareitnews. com/news/nurses-not-happy-hospital-ehrs.

32. Dowding DW, Turley M, Garrido T. The impact of an electronic health record on nurse sensitive patient outcomes: an interrupted time series analysis. *J Am Med Inform Assoc.* 2012;19:615–620.

33. Manca DP. Do electronic medical records improve quality of care? Yes. *Can Fam Physician.* 2015;61:846–847.

34. Kern LM, Barron Y, Dhopeshwarkar RV, et al. Electronic health records and ambulatory quality of care. *J Gen Intern Med.* 2013;28:496–503.

35. Bowles K, Hanlon A, Holland D, Potashnik S, Topaz M. Impact of discharge planning decision support on time to readmission among older adult medical patients. *Prof Case Manag.* 2014;19(1):1–10.

36. Higgins TC, Crosson J, et al. *Using Health Information Technology to Support Quality Improvement in Primary Care.* Agency for Healthcare Research and Quality, U.S. Department of Health and Human Services; March 2015 . AHRQ Publication No. 15-00031-EF.

37. Westbrook JI, Duffield C, Li L, Creswick NJ. How much time do nurses have for patients? A longitudinal study quantifying hospital nurses' patterns of task time distribution and interactions with health professionals. *BMC Health Serv Res.* 2011;11:319–331.

38. National Institute for Health and Care Excellence (NICE). Medicines Optimisation: The Safe and Effective Use of Medicines to Enable the Best Possible Outcomes. 2015; NICE Guideline #5.

39. Redman DD. Reducing medication errors in the OR. *AORN J.* 2017;105:106–109.

40. Morgan P, Everett CM, Hing E. Time spent with patients by physicians, nurse practitioners, and physician assistants in community health. *Healthc (Amst).* 2014;2:232–237.

41. Insurance Institute for Highway Safety. (online) http://www.iihs.org/iihs/topics/laws/safetybeltuse/mapbeltenforcement.

42. U.S. National Highway Traffic Safety Administration. 2014. (online) https://crashstats.nhtsa.dot.gov/Api/Public/ViewPublication/812262.

43. National Cancer Institute. Breast Cancer. (online) https://www.cancer.gov/types/breast/ibc-fact-sheet.

44. Ferguson MA. Office evaluation of rectal bleeding. *Clin Colon Rectal Surg.* 2005;18:249–254.

45. Strickberger SA, Benson DW, Biaggioni I, et al. AHA/ACCF Scientific Statement on the evaluation of syncope. *Circulation.* 2006;113:316–327.

CHAPTER 8

Interprofessional Education and Collaborative Practice

Michelle R. Troseth, MSN, RN, FNAP, FAAN,
Tracy Christopherson, MS, BAS, RRT

Our colleague, Dr. Peter Edelstein, knew who to come to for a discussion of the growing focus on **Interprofessional Education (IPE) and Collaborative Practice (CP)** (together, **IPECP**) and in appreciating the increasing importance and critical role that IPECP must play in navigating the healthcare reform revolution with the goal of achieving sustainable, high value healthcare. We hope at this point that you are celebrating that a *physician* (and a *surgeon,* of all things!) is asking a *nurse* and a *respiratory therapist* to pen the chapter on the ultimate *lifesaver* to survive *The Perfect Healthcare Reform Storm.* Together, we two authors of this chapter have decades of experience in advancing interprofessional care in academic, community, and rural practice settings and most recently have focused our mission-driven work towards **IPE** and bridging the gap between academia and clinical practice. You will never meet two more passionate people to share (and *shout from the rooftops—or perhaps from the deck of a cruise ship, in keeping with the nautical theme) that the future is all about interprofessional education and collaborative practice!*

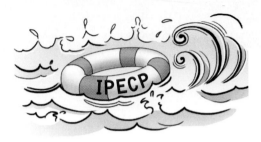

Interprofessional Education and Collaborative Practice

Throughout this book, Peter has provided you with the big picture regarding the *Perfect Healthcare Reform Storm.* In this chapter, we'll review how IPE and collaborative practice represent two of the major shifts in thinking that are foundational in the new paradigm.

IPECP is not a new concept. For over 40 years, there has been an awareness that "team-based care" is essential to the consistent delivery of quality care and a necessity for health profession students in preparation for collaborative team practice. IPE, according to the World Health Organization,[1] occurs when *students of two or more professions learn with, from, and about each other to enable effective collaboration and improve health outcomes;* and IPECP occurs when *multiple health workers from different professional backgrounds work together with patients, families, carers [caregivers], and communities to deliver the highest quality of care.*

> IPECP occurs when *multiple health workers from different professional backgrounds work together with patients, families, carers [caregivers], and communities to deliver the highest quality of care.*

Advancing IPECP is multifaceted and complex and, by and large, healthcare and academic institutions over the last several decades have not had the necessary guidance or infrastructures in place to support IPECP in a sustainable manner. As a result, the majority of the current healthcare workforce has been trained as *individual professionals,* within separate educational programs, resulting in *fragmentation of knowledge and healthcare practices.* Having been trained in isolation, the majority of today's providers are unprepared to successfully collaborate in a true team environment within our complex healthcare settings.[2]

Unfortunately, the unidisciplinary fashion in which allied health professionals are educated (and in which providers' beliefs and values are *hardwired* around their own individual professional domain) significantly influences their ability to adapt to new ways of thinking and practicing as a team.[3] In addition, organizational culture and infrastructures within the healthcare and academic environments have perpetuated the isolation of health professions and professionals.[3]

The best way to bring to life these troubling patient care realities is to share some of our own personal experiences with you.

PEARL

Unless we address how disciplines are prepared for collaborative practice in academia, we will not achieve IPECP, nor will it be sustainable.

The Voice of the Nurse

This year marks my (Michelle's) 40th year in healthcare. Wow! While I try not to be shocked by that fact, I also realize it brings 40 years of incredible experience and lessons learned that offer wisdom and hope to students and clinicians who desire to practice together in highly collaborative environments. Like so many clinicians, my advocacy for interprofessional collaborative practice came from a personal experience that greatly impacted my career path and life's work in the turbulent waters of healthcare.

As a new graduate nurse, I began my practice in an intensive care unit (ICU) of a community hospital. Despite the controversy of beginning a nursing practice in such an intense environment, I had proven myself to be an excellent nursing student and had brought real work experience to my goal of becoming the best critical care nurse I could be. Having worked in this same ICU as a student, I had already formed some strong relationships with other care providers. The support and mentoring offered by the ICU nursing management and experienced ICU nurses could not have been better.

In this environment, I became the primary nurse for a patient named Anna. Anna suffered from a chronic lung disease and had been on a mechanical ventilator with a tracheotomy tube for a long time. I think it is fair to say that Anna and I developed a special connection. While I was never really able to put my finger on what that connection was, I suppose Anna reminded me of my grandmother (and, in my mind, I could actually *see my grandmother* at different times while caring for Anna). At the start of my 7 PM–to–7 AM shift, I would walk by Anna's room. She would be sitting up in bed, a fan blowing her wild, white hair about her face, and she would wave at me. She would then use hand gestures while staring at me with her piercing blue eyes.

"Are *you* taking care of *me* tonight?" her eyes asked, simultaneously conveying *"please say yes!"*

Yes, we had a special connection. We had been through a lot together. In the long time Anna was in the ICU, she had suffered a cardiopulmonary arrest, and I had assisted her through many invasive and painful procedures. Despite her troubled physical body, her spirit always lit up the room. She seemed to accept her current reality of life as it was, and always smiled that incredible smile, with those baby blue eyes that radiated wisdom and love to all who entered her room. She became a "favorite patient" of mine and also of a respiratory therapist colleague, Amy. Together, Amy and I worked collaboratively over weeks caring for Anna's debilitating respiratory status while at the same time tending to the person, the human being, beyond the tracheostomy.

One night while caring for Anna, I had the responsibility to prepare her for a surgical procedure that was to take place first thing the next morning. We had completed all the necessary pre-surgical steps and paperwork (this was in the days of the pre-electronic health record) and were waiting for the transport team to come and wheel her off to the operating room (OR). I vividly remember standing at the nurse's station preparing for shift report and waiting for the OR transport team to show up when Anna's cardiac monitor began alarming. Her heart rhythm had suddenly changed. I did a quick assessment, which revealed no significant changes in her status. I was baffled by this threatening rhythm suddenly presenting itself to me. It was different from anything I had learned about in my training. When the transport team arrived, I informed them they were not to take Anna until we knew what was going on with her heart. Just then, a medical resident, Dr. S, walked through the ICU doors. Dr. S was freshly showered, and his wet hair was combed back. He wore his starched, white lab coat and he held a cup of steaming-hot coffee in a white Styrofoam cup. I thought, "Thank God Dr. S is here," for I had great respect for this physician. He was extremely intelligent, and often we would spend hours at the nurse's station on his on-call nights, where he would teach us about various medical conditions.

There was no doubt among the nurses that Dr. S was an excellent medical resident and had a very bright future as a physician.

I quickly approached Dr. S, who already had a patient chart open as he prepared for his morning ICU rounds. Armed with the cardiac strips and other important data, I explained Anna's situation, and that the OR team was waiting for our medical evaluation of the patient before transporting her from the ICU. I knew he knew Anna well from her lengthy ICU stay. Dr. S. looked at the strip and muttered under his breath, "It's MAT." Quickly, I am scanned my brain for anything I could recall from nursing school or my EKG class on "MAT." Nothing! So ... I asked, "What is MAT, and what does it mean for Anna right now, given that she is scheduled to go to the OR?"

Dr. S looked directly at me and said with distain in his voice, *"Go look it up. I am not here to spoon-feed the nurses."*

At that moment, I felt shock, disbelief, and ... outrage. This was no longer about the patient; this was about something else getting in the way of providing the safest, highest quality care for our patient. This was a *voluntarily lack of provider collaboration* smacking me right in the face ... *and it stung!*

The sequence of the events that followed that morning is not as clear to me as the events leading up to Dr. S's harsh words. I recall getting the charge nurse involved and advocating for an anesthesiologist (or some physician, *any* physician) to evaluate Anna's situation prior to her being shipped off to surgery. I told the oncoming nurse to stand guard over Anna's bed, keeping the OR transport team at bay until we had "medical clearance" for her to leave the ICU and undergo her scheduled procedure.

After turning Anna's care over to the next nurse, I found myself in the staff lounge ... and in tears.

My tears were not because I felt sorry for myself or even about my humiliation in front of my colleagues at the nurses' station. My tears were not because I had never learned about or was not able to recognize multifocal atrial tachycardia (MAT) by glancing at an EKG monitor strip. My tears were for this first experience of a *disconnect between two committed professionals caring for a patient* and for the incredible risk that such a disconnect (an entirely avoidable disconnect) represented for our patient's health. Tears were also flowing down my face because I respected this particular physician's medical knowledge and diagnostic abilities so much that I knew the patient couldn't be in better hands, and yet he was the person who let down both Anna and me.

Now for the "rest of the story." Three years went by, and I grew in my experience as a critical care nurse, eventually assuming a leadership role in the same ICU. During that time, Dr. S successfully completed his medical residency. Yes, we had many interactions, but neither of us could deny that things were "different" since that day when Anna's heart rhythm had changed. Dr. S's "spoon-feed" comment always lay underneath the surface of whatever we were doing at the moment.

Right before Dr. S graduated from his residency and left the hospital to begin his own medical practice in a different city, he sought me out. Much to my surprise, he said, "Before I leave, I owe you an apology." We both knew instantly to what he was referring. He went on to share quite candidly that the events of that morning had bothered him for 3 years. *Three years!* He knew how he had acted, what he had so harshly said, was wrong, and he did not want to leave without clearing the slate and offering his sincere apology. By then, he had watched me practice the science and art of nursing for 3 years, and he considered me "one of the best." I told him how much I held him in the deepest regard as a physician, and my frustration those many years ago had come from that place. He promised me he would always listen to nurses and build a very collaborative practice as he set out to begin his new journey in the private internal medicine world.

Dr. S's apology (even 3 years later) taught me that despite our titles and our traditions, we providers are all connected at a very human level, and *we should never deny that wonderful reality.* In fact, only when that pure and simple truth is embraced can we honestly make a real difference in our own and each other's lives, including the lives of our patients, and meaningfully contribute to a true interprofessional approach to patient care.

Twenty years later, I shared this story while participating in an interprofessional workshop. My group's assignment was to "name the story." A physician in the group quietly named it as a *"Defining Moment."* Immediately, I realized just what a defining moment those minutes long ago in the ICU standing at Anna's bedside really was for me and for my healthcare career journey. It lit a fire in my belly, a drive to serve as a role model and advocate for interprofessional collaborative practice.

Shortly after Dr. S left our hospital, I, too, moved on to work at another hospital that had recently committed to developing a professional practice model intentionally designed to *create the best place to give and receive care.* I also went to graduate school where I focused my Master's Thesis on *"Nurse-Physician Collaboration and Nurse Satisfaction."* My research validated that a higher level of collaborative practice perceived by nurses and physicians resulted in greater satisfaction among nurses.[4] There I had it … my long-standing hypothesis that the more we providers collaborate, the greater our own professional satisfaction, was now statistically proven and backed by evidence-based data!

Why is this important? Think back to the first chapter of this book: we are all in a health profession not only to improve patient care, but to improve our personal and professional satisfaction as well.

> The more we collaborate, the greater our own professional satisfaction.

One of my greatest surprises in writing my Master's thesis came through a thesis committee member who was not a clinician, but a PhD Professor from the Sociology Department. He shared that, for the first time, he really understood that nurses were not "physician extenders," but that nurses had a unique scope-of-practice that functioned both independently and interdependently with the activities of physicians. Exactly right! *Nurses and allied health professionals are not "physician extenders,"* and we are poised to lead (we *must lead*) the current healthcare reform efforts if our society is to "right the ship" and create IPE and collaborative practice environments across the continuum of care.

The Voice of the Respiratory Therapist

Like Michelle, I (Tracy) can hardly believe I have been in healthcare for so long … over 30 years. Of course, both of us were only toddlers when we entered our respective professions!

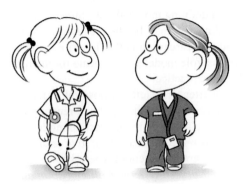

These clinicians just keep
getting younger and younger!

I have had many experiences and learned many lessons working as a respiratory therapist and leader in healthcare. Collectively these experiences have led me to be an advocate for IPECP, and I have been fortunate to have spent the majority of my career working with healthcare organizations to develop collaborative practice environments. I feel fortunate to have shared these meaningful journeys with other healthcare providers and stakeholders and to learn with them, from them, and about them. The road to IPECP is truly a journey, so I'd like to share with you an experience in the hope that it helps you as you travel along your own practice path.

In the early 1990s, I was working at a 529-bed teaching hospital as a staff respiratory therapist. I had previously worked in a small community hospital and had chosen to join the staff at this particular institution thinking that their reputation for advanced respiratory practices would offer me the best opportunity to develop my skills and grow as a professional. But 6 years later, I was frustrated. I was not practicing at the top of my professional abilities (I say this rather than "at the top of my license," because at the time, respiratory therapists were not licensed in this state). I knew I had more to offer the patients for whom I cared for, yet I felt powerless to practice at a higher level, and what I was providing in the way of patient care was clearly not well regarded by most of the physicians, nurses, and other members of the provider team. Thus, both my patients were getting short-changed, and my own professional satisfaction was suffering.

With regard to collaborative teamwork, it was a struggle. The relationships across the professions were hierarchical. At the top were the doctors (the Gods, as Peter previously described them); then came the nurses (maybe we should call them the Angels!); followed by everyone else. The rest of the allied health professionals were only rarely even referred to by their specific provider designations; rather, they were simply lumped together as "non-nurses" or "ancillary services" (today, we're grouped into "allied health professionals"). Even today, every time I hear this term it makes the hair on the back of my neck stand up (it is probably the same for you when you hear your professional self lumped together in this bucket term). For the most part, we were working *alongside* each other but not really working *together.* I can't paint a totally grim picture; indeed, there were a few units in the hospital where the relationships across the provider team were more collaborative and where each profession, mine included, were mutually respected and relied upon. The problem was that these interprofessional team environments were few and far between.

Then the best thing that could have happened, happened: *patients started to complain* as they began to experience the downside of their providers' lack of collaborative care. Patients complained about all the duplication and repetition in their care. They complained about the lack of coordination in their care. Patients complained that they were repeatedly asked the same questions over and over again, leading them to openly respond, *"Do you people ever talk to each other?!"*

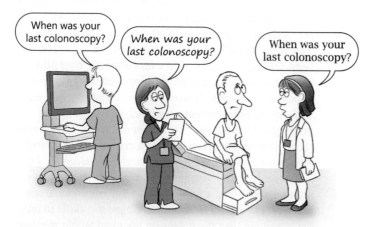

PEARL

Interprofessional practice today is largely being driven from patient expectations and their desire for coordinated, consistent, collaborative, and high quality care.

Luckily, our patients' voices were heard, and leadership asked us to address their concerns. As a participant in a subsequent initiative to explore how our respiratory therapists, physical therapists, occupational therapists, speech language pathologists, dietitians, and social workers could enhance our communication and collaboration in delivering care, I supported our first step: to gain an honest understanding of our current practice environment reality. It didn't take long for us to collectively realize that the patients' complaints and concerns were well founded (can you believe it?). We were working in silos. We were asking the same questions and, even though each of us captured the responses to those questions in our documentation (behind our own separate tab silo in the paper chart), we were failing to look at (let alone consider the clinical impact of) what each other was documenting.

I'm sure you are totally shocked, right? *Not!* This provider silo phenomenon is unfortunately still all too prevalent in hospitals all over the country today.

As a team, we began to explore the use of documentation tools that empowered all providers' mutual visibility, reducing the duplication of efforts that were reducing our efficiency and annoying (and worrying) our patients. It soon became clear that we needed to learn more about each other's professions, the services we each provided, and how our activities and professional perspectives were communicated to the entire team. It was during this process improvement I experienced one of the most significant "Aha!" moments of my career, one which forever changed how I perceived both my own practice and the practices of the other professionals with whom I worked with every day. You see, I thought I knew what nurses did. After all, I have been practicing side by side with nurses for over 10 years. I had witnessed nurses administering medications, assessing patient's vital signs, dressing wounds, and carrying out a variety of other patient care tasks, so I felt I had a pretty good handle on what nurses did. What I had never recognized and appreciated was a critical nursing function: *nurses are skilled at diagnosing and addressing the human response.* In fact, I was shocked to realize that I knew nothing about this, a foundation of the professional nursing practice. I had always attributed diagnostic skills to only the physician. But the nurses on my team taught me that the *nursing diagnosis,* the nurses' professional ability to assess a patient's or patient's family's response, experience, and concern over an actual or potential health problem *is a critical patient care function.*

If you are not a nurse, how well do you honestly understand this and other critical aspects of nursing's practice? *Do you know what you don't know?* As I said, I certainly didn't appreciate all of the unique and significant aspects of successful nursing care. And it made me ask, *what don't they know about me as a respiratory therapist?* Was this why I wasn't feeling respected, why I wasn't being empowered to support patients to my fullest abilities?

> The nurses on my team taught me that the *nursing diagnosis,* the nurses' professional ability to assess a patient's or patient's family's response, experience, concern over an actual or potential health problem, *is a critical patient care function.*

This is where IPECP must begin. By asking yourself and other members of your provider "team," *what do you know and what do you not know about each other's professional training, skills, competencies, responsibilities, focus, goals?* You must move away from the traditional view of other providers (the view I originally had) in which you see other professions only as the services they obviously provide. Learn as I did to find what is below the surface, to *appreciate the critical thinking and decision making capabilities that may be unique to certain providers and which can enhance the care provided the patient by the entire team.*

This "Aha!" moment was the spark that ignited my personal and professional passion for advancing scope-of-practice clarity across the healthcare team and which ultimately led to my commitment to IPE and collaborative practice.

> Find what is below the surface … *appreciate the critical thinking and decision making capabilities that may be unique to certain providers and which can enhance the care provided the patient by the entire team.*

Nor was I alone in incorrectly assuming I understood my professional colleagues. Through intentional efforts, we began to understand the significant impact that attaining clarity on each team member's scope-of-practice would be both on our patients and on our own professional activities and satisfaction.

I now have had the privilege to co-lead (with two nursing colleagues) an initiative across a large healthcare

 PEARL

A cornerstone of IPECP is *clarity on scope-of-practice,* allowing each discipline to practice both independently and interdependently to meet the needs and values of every patient and family, guided by evidence-based information.

PEARL

The more clarity provided nurses and allied health professionals have on their colleagues' scopes-of-practice, the more they can *lead the way in significantly driving healthcare reform.*

consortium aimed at identifying and developing tools, processes, and infrastructures that support the advancement of "interdisciplinary practice" (as it was called back then). Again, *the first step in successfully advancing IPECP was to first understand each other's scope-of-practice.* This requires us to *dive deep* to truly understand where our practices are unique, where our skills and responsibilities overlap, and, most importantly, *where our skills and responsibilities empower one another to advance the value of our own patient care activities.*

That we providers often erroneously believe we understand each other's capabilities (to the detriment of our patients) was beautifully summed up by another respiratory therapist who participated in our healthcare consortium initiative: "I expected colleagues to know what I do, but I found it hard to put into words." If we are not able to articulate to others our scope-of-practice, how can we expect them to understand what we do (and hope to do)? Thus, an important activity is to try and *clearly articulate out loud* (as it is always perfect when said in your head, but out loud is something different!) your scope-of-practice; that is, your training and experience, your skills and capabilities, and your patient care responsibilities and goals.

Trust me. You'll likely be surprised by how difficult this is to do the first time. But with a little practice, you'll succeed, and when the time comes (and you should make it come sooner rather than later), you will successfully share this new knowledge with your provider teammates, empowering them and benefitting your patients.

> An important activity is to try and *clearly articulate out loud* your scope-of-practice; that is, your training and experience, your skills and capabilities, and your patient care responsibilities and goals.

While it is critical that you and your interprofessional colleagues work together to create clear scope-of-practice descriptions, it is the process itself (even more than the concrete outcomes) that most significantly impacts team bonding and future collaboration. That is, *simply engaging in open, honest, meaningful conversations with healthcare peers within and across our professions was enormously beneficial and impactful in changing our thinking and our patient care behaviors.* One such interaction captures the essence of such a team building experience:

I was working on a medical-surgical floor, assigned
to a patient with an acute exacerbation of his chronic
obstructive pulmonary disease (COPD). His breathing
difficulties were significant, requiring me to assess him
and administer respiratory treatments every 2 hours. I
clearly recognized that this was a pivotal period in his care,
given our mutual goal to avoid his needing intubation and
mechanical ventilator support. Coincidentally, the timing
of his breathing treatments coincided with the delivery of
his meals, so he had either just finished eating or food was
delivered during his respiratory treatments. I had never paid
much attention to what patients were served on their meal
trays, but on this day, for some reason, I noticed a pattern:
each of his meals included multiple, small containers of ice
cream, along with some liquids, but little else.

Now, first you have to know that *I love ice cream,* so I
was eyeing those containers a bit enviously! As I prepared
to administer yet another breathing treatment, he finished
his evening meal.

"I noticed that you have ice cream on all your meal trays,"
I commented. "You must really like ice cream!"

"Well, yes I do," he replied with a little smile. "But I eat
ice cream because I haven't really been able to eat much
else over the past couple of months."

I stared at him, puzzled. "Why is that?"

"Because," he replied, "every time I try to eat anything
solid, I can't swallow it and I choke."

I was stunned. "So," I probed further, "are you telling me
that *you've been eating only ice cream for the past few
months?*"

"Yep," he nodded.

As a respiratory therapist, I appreciated the importance
of adequate nutritional intake in maintaining the health
of patients suffering from chronic conditions, such as
this gentleman with COPD, so his comments were a
big, waving, red flag. If all he was eating was ice cream
and liquids, I immediately realized, then nutritional
depletion may well have contributed to his current COPD
exacerbation. Furthermore, if his nutritional status wasn't
rapidly and adequately addressed, my patient would have
difficulty avoiding intubation, let alone returning to a
stable respiratory state. And there was more: I realized

that his description of choking when attempting to eat solid foods might well represent a swallowing dysfunction that would also need to be evaluated and addressed.

Suddenly I thought back to my recent conversations with other members of our provider team. The scope-of-practice for our dietitian and our speech language pathologist came to mind, and I immediately consulted these colleagues, sharing with them our patient's history and current status.

I have to be honest in admitting that before being engaged in our interprofessional team building initiative, I probably would have just passed off my conversation with this COPD patient as nothing more than chit-chat, because *these seemingly non-respiratory problems were not within my scope-of-practice; furthermore, even had I become concerned, I would likely have felt that there was nothing I could do to address them.* I'm not proud of this reality, but it's the truth. And I encourage you to be honest with yourself and ask the tough questions:

- Do I focus *only on patient care issues that fall within my own scope-of-practice*?
- Do I truly, honestly *understand the breadth and depth of what other providers caring for my patients offer? Their skills? Their responsibilities?*
- Do I feel *empowered to reach out to other providers* when a potential clinical issue outside of my scope-of-practice arises?
- In fact, do I even *pursue potential patient issues that fall outside of my experience, knowledge, skills, and responsibilities?*

Our patients are more than respiratory problems, abdominal pains, fevers. They must be seen as *whole human beings whose care must be interprofessional, collaborated, and empowered by frequent, open communication in an environment that encourages providers to ask questions, raise concerns, offer input.* As my experience exemplified, our *patients don't always reveal critical information directly to the specific professional best suited to address the problem.* As members of the healthcare team, we must be each other's eyes and ears. We must broaden the lens through which we assess and care for our patients, allowing every provider to pick up on any critical pieces of information, facilitating involvement of the right provider resources whenever necessary.

It is this sense of collaboration, of trust, of "being on the same page" in terms of patient care, that drives better outcomes (both clinical and financial). It is an environment of open communication, freedom to question, and mutual support that empowers the best patient care. This is the foundation on which a deeper understanding of one another's scope-of-practice is built.

> *Simply engaging in open, honest, meaningful conversations with healthcare peers within and across our professions was enormously beneficial and impactful in changing our thinking and our patient care behaviors.*

Another important lesson learned during our team's interprofessional care discussions was that many of our professional processes-of-care were shared by most or all of our different team members. This realization led us to conclude that if the documentation tools we utilized reflected these processes-of-care commonalities, we could empower collaborative patient care by utilizing the same health information technology (HIT) solutions; that is, *our shared HIT solutions could facilitate the integration of our interprofessional care by providing mutual access to and communication and coordination of patient care.* I am proud to say that our team's work was integrated in our systems' clinical practice model and is now utilized as part of the electronic health record (EHR) in hundreds of healthcare organizations.

> *Our shared HIT solutions could facilitate the integration of our interprofessional care by providing mutual access to and communication and coordination of patient care.*

Although my story is from 25 years ago, it remains incredibly relevant today, as the patient care issues we faced are still prevalent: the rarity of truly interprofessional care delivery. Allied health professionals, nurses, physicians, and others continue duplicating services, asking patients the same questions over and over, and working in clinical isolation. The truth is, there is no one individual, healthcare discipline, or clinical department that can alone deliver the quality of care that Peter has encouraged throughout this book. *It will take a team of providers* truly working together to integrate care in the collaborative manner that provides our patients and our healthcare system the greatest value. And again, at the heart of this interprofessional care model is team clarity on each provider's scope-of-practice and an environment of open communication and shared goals.

So, when was the last time you had a real conversation with another professional about what they do? About their patient care focus? Their sense of their responsibilities? What assumptions do you have about the other professions and the services they can provide (be honest here, as you likely know only a fraction of what your colleagues offer, just as they likely grossly underestimate your capabilities)? *Look for opportunities to share* your skills and knowledge and goals with other providers. *Seek to understand* the tremendous expertise of those with whom you work on a daily basis. *Take the lead* to empower collaborative patient care. Your patients will benefit, and so will you.

One last thing. You have probably noticed that physicians were not present in my stories. At the time that these activities took place, physicians didn't feel a sense of urgency to participate in "interprofessional care." We respected their feelings and made the conscious decision to move forward without them, anticipating that once we created a collaborative team environment, we would be ready when they were ready to join in. Well, *that time is now!* So, physicians, ready or not, here we come! As Peter has shared earlier in this book, *we are all Providers,* and if we are to realize meaningful healthcare reform, if we are to consistently deliver high quality, cost-efficient patient care, if we are to achieve the Triple Aim, we must understand each other's scope-of-practice, we must communicate, we must collaborate.

We must work together.

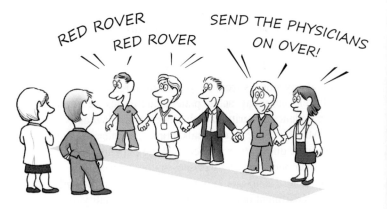

It's About the Team

Having worked with allied health professionals and healthcare organizations across North America for over 20 years, we can safely say that the stories we've shared are not unique to us, but are representative of the experiences had by many of the professionals working in healthcare organizations today. The good news is that IPECP momentum has been building over the past decade, fueled by the changing healthcare landscape Peter has described and also informed by the lessons learned over the previous 30 years. We next wish to share some of the significant developments that have occurred both nationally and internationally, which fill us with the hope that this time it sails, the IPECP ship will stay afloat and carry us through the healthcare reform storm and into a sustainable collaborative future.

The Call for Nurses to Lead the Way

While it is about the interprofessional team, there have been national initiatives that have focused on the role of nursing, encouraging nurses to be more engaged and to empower nurses to *toss the traditional healthcare model overboard!* As a continuation of the *Voice of the Nurse,* I (Michelle) will share some significant national initiatives and explain why mobilizing *nursing as a profession* is critically important to navigating the healthcare reform storm as well as to further advancing IPECP.

Nurses are the largest healthcare workforce in the United States.[5] With more than 3 million nurses working the front lines of patient care, these providers can and must play a critical role in helping realize the objectives set forth in the 2009 HITECH Act and the 2010 Affordable Care Act. In addition to my "day job," I have been actively engaged in two national efforts whose goals were to (1) mobilize the US nursing workforce to embrace technology and informatics competencies *and* (2) lead change and advance health across the country. These two national efforts are the **Technology Informatics Guiding Education Reform (TIGER) Initiative**[6] and the Institute of Medicine Report (2010) **The Future of Nursing: Leading Change, Advancing Health.**[7]

Let me start with TIGER, an initiative that was ultimately joined by over 1500 nurse volunteers across the country. The roots of the now decade old TIGER crusade began as a result of the lack of acknowledgment of the significant roles nurses and allied health professionals need to play in digitalizing the US healthcare system. *Duh, right?* Nurses and nurse advocates recognized the opportunity for *nurses to lead the way.* And indeed, that is exactly what happened. Here is the true story of how TIGER got started:

In early 2004, US President George W. Bush declared the *Decade for Health Information Technology*[8] and created the Office of the National Coordinator of Health Information Technology. In May 2004, Secretary of Health and Human Services, Tommy Thompson, appointed Dr. David Brailer as the first National Health Information Technology Coordinator. This was an exciting time for allied health professionals committed to the transformational role that HIT could play in substantially improving patient safety and care efficiency as well as driving other health reform efforts. In July 2004, Dr. Brailer convened the first national Health Information Technology Summit in Washington, D.C., and launched the *Framework for Strategic Action*[9] to provide US citizens with the benefits of EHRs within a 10-year period. And guess what? *The only clinical provider mentioned as a critical stakeholder in this aggressive initiative was the physician. No mention of nurses. No mention of any other allied health professionals.*

That the ship was headed directly towards an enormous iceberg was obvious. And so nursing leaders across the country put out a major *SOS distress call...*

Leaders in nursing keenly felt the *sense of urgency* to initiate a grassroots effort on the heels of this initial physician-focused HIT summit. In effect, the summit gave birth to a movement that would ensure nurses were at the table and recognized as key stakeholders and advocates in the strategic and tactical integration of health information technologies into the nation's healthcare delivery systems and academic training programs.

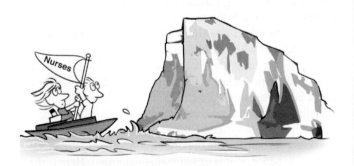

In 2005, I joined a diverse group of national nurse leaders at the Johns Hopkins School of Nursing to delineate the vision of TIGER and to identify necessary actions to achieve that vision. In October 2006, I served as Program Chair of the TIGER Summit, which was entirely focused on creating movement towards consensus on a 10-year vision and a 3-year action plan to empower nurses to *lead the way* in integrating technology into daily practice.

Here's what the over 100 nurses at the summit quickly realized: *our vision and action plan needed to be viewed through an interprofessional lens.* We realized that designing technology and systems in a nursing-only silo would fail to deliver meaningful, sustainable healthcare for patients or for clinicians.

Over 10 years after its birth, TIGER[10] is now an interprofessional community of the **Health Information Management Systems Society (HIMSS).** The TIGER Virtual Learning Environment (VLE) is used by numerous interprofessional colleagues to leverage HIT in the advancement of interprofessional learning and patient care. (*Please hear my roar* and tap the TIGER resources for tools to advance opportunities for nurses and allied health professionals to lead with technology!)

Many nurses also engaged in the second national effort, their testimonies and input helping to shape the *Institute of Medicine (IOM) Report on the Future of Nursing* (the most downloaded report in IOM history). The report identified a number of barriers that prevent nurses from effectively responding to the rapidly changing healthcare settings and evolving healthcare system. These barriers must be overcome to ensure that nurses are well positioned to lead change and advance health and healthcare value improvement.

In 2008, the Robert Wood Johnson Foundation (RWJF) and the IOM launched a 2-year initiative to respond to the need to assess and transform the nursing profession. The IOM appointed the Committee on the RWJF Initiative on the Future of Nursing, the purpose of which was to make recommendations for an action-oriented "blueprint" describing the future of nursing. Through its deliberations, the committee developed four key recommendations:

1. Nurses should practice to the full extent of their education and training.
2. Nurses should achieve higher levels of education and training through an improved education system that promotes seamless academic progression.

3. Nurses should be full partners with physicians and other allied healthcare professionals in redesigning healthcare in the United States.
4. Effective workforce planning and policy making require better data collection and information infrastructure.

Being a "full partner" requires that leadership and interprofessional competencies be applied *within and across the nursing profession* and in collaboration with other health professions. It calls for the recognition that *we all must be accountable for our own contributions in delivering high-quality care while working collaboratively together.* This is the entire premise behind interprofessional collaborative practice. The IOM report has also moved to reduce scope-of-practice barriers for advanced practice nurses and increased the number of doctoral-prepared and BSN-prepared nurses by 2020.

> *Nurses should be full partners, with physicians and other allied healthcare professionals, in redesigning healthcare in the United States.*

National and International Initiatives to Advance Interprofessional Education and Collaborative Practice

In 2000 and 2001, the IOM released two important reports: *To Err is Human*[11] and *Crossing the Quality Chasm.*[12] These reports heightened the awareness regarding the number of preventable medical errors occurring on a daily basis and the need for a redesigned healthcare delivery system which includes improved teamwork, collaboration, and communication across the health professions. In 2003, the IOM released a third report, *Health Professions Education: A Bridge to Quality.*[2] This report represents the strategies and actions identified during the Health Professions Education Summit aimed at redesigning health professions education in both academic and practice settings. To prepare allied health professionals in meeting the new demands of a redesigned healthcare system, a set of five core competencies were identified for allied health professions education, including[2 (pp45-56)]:

1. Providing patient-centered care
2. Working in interdisciplinary teams

3. Employing evidence-based practice
4. Applying quality improvement
5. Utilizing informatics

The competencies associated with *patient-centered care* focus attention on *engaging with patients and families in ways that support their unique needs and values,* considering their preferences, supporting coordinated care across the continuum, educating patients and families, and advocating for actions that lead to improved health. The following three words best describe the competency of *working in interdisciplinary teams for the shared purpose of delivering dependable care:*

1. Communicate
2. Integrate
3. Collaborate

Employing evidence-based practice competency provides for nurses and allied health professionals to actively combine research outcomes with their own clinical knowledge and skills while taking into account patient values, all aimed at decision making which achieves the best possible results for the patient. *Applying quality improvement* emphasizes *the development of knowledge and skills,* allowing us to learn from and utilize our experiences along with processes and infrastructures to develop and evaluate new standards of care delivery. Last but not least, the competency of *utilizing informatics* addresses the need to leverage health information technology in ways that enhance communication, reduce errors, and support clinical decision making at the moment of care delivery. The release of this IOM report and the competencies cited have prompted new initiatives in both academic and practice settings and generated new momentum for an already 30-year-old concept.

Since the release of the IOM report in 2003, several groups (both nationally and internationally) have worked to further define IPE and collaborative practice and to develop core competencies applicable across the health professions. In 2006, the Canadian Interprofessional Health Collaborative (CIHC) began a 2-year Health Canada funded initiative aimed at building a national collaborative of partners to advance the field and implementation of *Interprofessional Education for Collaborative Patient-Centered Practice.*[13] In 2010, the WHO released the *Framework for Action on Interprofessional Education and Collaborative Practice.*[1] This report provided a clear definition for "interprofessional education" and established what it means to have a "collaborative practice-ready

 PEARL

Several national and international initiatives and organizations are advancing the IPECP agenda, moving it from vision to reality. It is critical that nurses and allied health professionals are engaged to lead reform activities so that consistent, sustainable, high-value healthcare can be realized.

health work force." In 2010, the CIHC released *A National Interprofessional Competency Framework*[14] that has provided additional guidance on the development of competencies for IPE, and in May 2011, the Interprofessional Education Collaborative (IPEC) Expert Panel within the United States released the report, *Core Competencies for Interprofessional Collaborative Practice.*[15] IPEC included representatives from six national associations of health professions schools, including dentistry, nursing, medicine, osteopathic medicine, and pharmacy, to inform curriculum development, support the advancement of team-based care, and enhance population outcomes. The expert panel drew from the work already done by the CIHC and the IOM. The core competencies were organized under four IPE competency domains:

1. Values and Ethics for Interprofessional Practice
2. Roles and Responsibilities for Collaborative Practice
3. Interprofessional Communication Practices
4. Interprofessional Teamwork and Team-based Practice

Each of these domains included a number of competencies developed with the intention that the competencies would support nursing and allied health professional education across the continuum from pre-licensure to practice. The competencies were kept broad enough to meet the unique needs of the profession, program, or institution. In IPEC's recent report, *Core Competencies for Interprofessional Collaborative Practice: 2016 Update,*[16] nine additional institutional members were included, representing podiatric medicine, physical therapy, occupational therapy, psychology, veterinary medicine, optometry, social work, physician assistants, and the schools of allied health professions. These core competencies have been embraced nationally and internationally and have been updated to more accurately reflect the current healthcare environment, the Triple Aim, and federally legislated healthcare reform (the Affordable Care Act, also known as the ACA and "ObamaCare"). Two notable changes include utilizing *Interprofessional Collaboration* as the central domain (instead of having four individual domains) and the integration of more specific population health competencies (in support of the Triple Aim). Under the Interprofessional Collaboration domain, there are now four core competencies and related sub competencies. The four core competencies include[16]:

1. Work with individuals of other professions to maintain a climate of mutual respect and shared values *(Values/ Ethics for Interprofessional Practice)*

2. Use the knowledge of one's own role and those of other professions to appropriately assess and address the healthcare needs of patients and to promote and advance the health of populations *(Roles/Responsibilities)*
3. Communicate with patients, families, communities, and professionals in health and other fields in a responsive and responsible manner that supports a team approach to the promotion and maintenance of health and the prevention and treatment of disease *(Interprofessional Communication)*
4. Apply relationship-building values and the principles of team dynamics to perform effectively in different team roles to plan, deliver, and evaluate patient/population-centered care and population health programs and policies that are safe, timely, efficient, effective, and equitable *(Teams and Teamwork)*

Organizations Advancing Interprofessional Education and Collaborative Practice

With the sweeping changes in healthcare delivery and the revitalized momentum around IPECP, a growing need for a national US center was recognized. In 2012, after the completion of a competitive process, the University of Minnesota was awarded the designation as the National Center for Interprofessional Practice and Education.[17] The Center is supported by funds from the Department of Health and Human Services, along with private foundations (such as the Josiah Macey Jr. Foundation, RWJF, and the Gordon and Betty Moore Foundation). The National Center serves as a coordinating body for the advancement of IPE and practice. The Center's efforts are focused on what they describe as "the Nexus."[18] The Nexus represents the relationship between practice settings where healthcare is delivered, health professions education, and the collaboration necessary to prepare the current and future healthcare workforce to achieve the Triple Aim. To support the implementation of IPECP, the Center offers a wide variety of resources, tools, and learning opportunities, along with access to communities of individuals who are engaged in advancing IPECP.[19] In addition, the Center uses a network of institutions and organizations involved in IPECP, and a data repository which gathers data and provides evidence of the effectiveness of IPE and collaborative practice.

National Academies of Practice

Because each of us is currently or ultimately affected by health policies (for good or bad), it is helpful to think about how allied health professionals can have an IMPACT on policy. Although each of our professional organizations is no doubt engaged in health policy advocacy, there is *one forum that solely focuses on health policy to advance interprofessional collaboration:* the National Academies of Practice (NAP).[20] NAP is a nonprofit organization founded in 1981 to advise governmental bodies on our healthcare system. Distinguished practitioners and scholars are elected by their peers from fourteen different health professions to join the only interprofessional group of healthcare practitioners and scholars dedicated to supporting affordable, accessible, coordinated, quality healthcare for all. (We encourage all of you who are— or might be—interested in advancing interprofessional collaborative practice in healthcare to join *the National Academies of Practice and/or align your organization in partnership with NAP.* The more voices we have, the stronger our collective voice is to integrate collaboration into the US healthcare delivery system!)

In April of 2016, NAP collaborated with other nationally funded organizations to create a formal Proclamation making the month of April *National Interprofessional Health Care Month.*[21] Thus, each year, April is a dedicated opportunity for all allied health professionals to come together and plan, act, and celebrate any and all efforts in leading new ways of learning and practicing together. So *mark your calendars!*

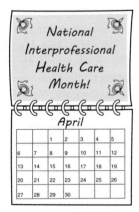

Moving Toward the *Quadruple Aim*

As our colleague Peter has pointed out, a major roadmap to reforming the US healthcare system is the Triple Aim. This chapter on advancing IPE and collaborative practice has a major emphasis on each discipline's scope-of-practice as well as on providing caregivers with a high level of work satisfaction through collaborative practice. We hope we have made the message clear that, in today's complex health environments, none of us can care for patients in isolation. We need a team-based approach, and we must focus on the *work life* of all healthcare providers, including nursing and allied health professionals. Decreased work satisfaction can lead to burnout and has an impact on the quality of care delivered to our patients. Recently, the issue of provider satisfaction has been raised (and is gaining momentum), begging the following question: should the Triple Aim actually be the *Quadruple Aim,* including "Care of Clinicians" (i.e., "*Improve the Clinician Experience*")?[22]

Here are some suggestions for enhancing both the individual provider's and care team's experience, while also improving the patient experience, delivering better clinical outcomes (for both individual patients and populations), and reducing the costs of care:

PEARL

Momentum is growing to shift to a "Quadruple Aim" that addresses the missing piece of *improved clinician experience.* This includes *all clinicians on the interprofessional care team.*

- *Decrease fragmentation and duplication of services* through the implementation of integrated care planning and documentation, allowing all team members to contribute and track patient care goals.
- *Educate on professional scopes-of-practice and implement systems empowering providers to practice at the top of their license.* Rotate designated "lead roles" in patient rounding, safety check-ins, etc., providing all team members with leadership experience.
- *Implement a partnership council infrastructure* to connect caregivers on the most important issues within their care environments and across their care system.
- *Introduce standardized, evidence-based practice tools, and resources* to decrease variability and offset human-based errors.

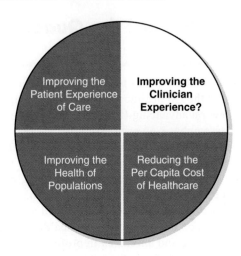

The Missing Fourth Aim?

Conclusions

IPE is one way to prepare the *future* healthcare workforce to function in collaborative, integrated teams that support achieving health and health system goals. However, *there is an interdependent relationship between interprofessional education and collaborative practice* (CP).[23-26] IPE students need to see CP role modeled by allied health professionals in the clinical setting.[23] To advance CP, the current health professions workforce needs to develop the knowledge, skills, attitudes, and competencies. The 2010 IOM report, *Redesigning Continuing Education in the Health Professions,*[27] emphasized that effective coordination and use of interprofessional teams of practitioners in the care setting requires practice and the development of a collaborative skill set that is *not routinely taught at other levels of health professions education.* As allied health professionals and leaders, we must be actively engaged in the efforts necessary to develop the healthcare cultures and environments that support CP. At the same time, we must be vigilant in taking action to prepare *both the current and future healthcare workforce* if CP is going to be sustained over time.

References

1. World Health Organization. *Framework for Action on Interprofessional Education & Collaborative Practice.* Geneva, Switzerland: WHO Press; 2010.
2. U.S. Institute of Medicine, Greiner A, Knebel E. *Health Professions Education: A Bridge to Quality.* Washington, DC: National Academy Press; 2003.

3. Christopherson T, Troseth M. Interprofessional education and practice: a 40-year old new trend experiencing rapid growth. *Comput Inform Nurs.* 2013;31(10):463–464.

4. Troseth M. Nurse-Physician Collaboration and Nurse Satisfaction. *Unpublished master's thesis*, Allendale, MI: Grand Valley State University; 1997.

5. U.S. Department of Health and Human Services, Health Resources and Services Administration, National Center for Health Workforce Analysis. *The Future of the Nursing Workforce: National- and State-Level Projections, 2012–2025.* Rockville, MD: HHS; 2014.

6. Technology Informatics Guiding Education Reform. *The TIGER Initiative: Evidence and Informatics Transforming Nursing: 3-Year Action Steps toward a 10-Year Vision* (online); 2007. http://www.aacn.nche.edu/education-resources/TIGER.pdf.

7. Committee on the Robert Wood Johnson Foundation Initiative on the Future of Nursing, at the Institute of Medicine, Robert Wood Johnson Foundation, & Institute of Medicine (U.S.). *The Future of Nursing: Leading Change, Advancing Health.* Washington, DC: National Academies Press; 2011.

8. Transforming Health Care. *The President's Health Information Technology Plan* (online); 2004. https://aspe.hhs.gov/system/files/pdf/122371/PresidentsHealthITPlan4-26-2004_0.pdf.

9. The Decade of Health Information Technology. *Delivering Consumer-centric and Information-rich Health Care Framework for Strategic Action* (online); 2004. http://www.providersedge.com/ehdocs/ehr_articles/the_decade_of_hit-delivering_customer-centric_and_info-rich_hc.pdf.

10. Healthcare Information and Management Systems Society. HIMSS Provides a Home for TIGER [Press Release] (online); 2014. http://www.himss.org/news/hims-provides-home-tiger.

11. Kohen LT, Corrigan J, Donaldson MS. *To Err Is Human: Building a Safer Health System.* Washington, DC: National Academy Press; 2000.

12. U.S. Institute of Medicine, Committee on Quality of Healthcare in America. *Crossing the Quality Chasm: A New Health System for the 21st Century.* Washington, DC: National Academy Press; 2001.

13. Gilbert JHV. Interprofessional education for collaborative, patient-centered practice. *Nurs Leadersh.* 2005;18(2):32–38.

14. Canadian Interprofessional Health Collaborative. *A National Interprofessional Competency Framework* (online); 2010. http://www.cihc.ca/resources/publications.

15. Interprofessional Education Collaborative Expert Panel. *Core Competencies for Interprofessional Collaborative Practice: Report of an Expert Panel* (online); 2011. http://www.aacn.nche.edu/education-resources/IPECReport.pdf.

16. Interprofessional Education Collaborative. *Core Competencies for Interprofessional Collaborative Practice: 2016 Update* (online); 2016. http://www.aacn.nche.edu/education-resources/IPEC-2016-Updated-Core-Competencies-Report.pdf.

17. Chen FM, Williams SD, Gardner DB. The case for a National Center for Interprofessional Practice and Education. *J Interprof Care.* 2013;27(5):356–357.

18. Brandt BF. Update on the U.S. national center for interprofessional practice and education. *J Interprof Care.* 2014;28(1):5–7.

19. University of Minnesota. *About the National Center* (online); 2017. https://nexusipe.org/informing/about-national-center.

20. *National Academies of Practice* (online); 2017. www.napractice.org.

21. National Academies of Practice. *National Interprofessional Health Care Month* (online); 2017. http://www.napractice.org/Advocacy/National-Interprofessional-Health-Care-Month.

22. Bodenheimer T, Sinsky C. From triple to quadruple aim: care of the patient requires care of the provider. *Ann Fam Med.* 2014;12(6):573–576.

23. Barr H. An anatomy of continuing interprofessional education. *J Contin Educ Health Prof.* 2009;29(3):147–150.

24. Cox M, Naylor M. *Transforming patient care: aligning interprofessional education with clinical practice redesign.* In: Larson T, ed. *Proceedings of a Conference Sponsored by the Josiah Macy Jr. Foundation January 2013* New York: Josiah Macy Jr. Foundation; 2013.

25. Greenfield D, Nugus P, Travagilia J, Braithwaite J. Auditing an organization's interprofessional learning and interprofessional practice: the interprofessional praxis audit framework (IPAF). *J Interprof Care.* 2010;24(4):436. 449.

26. Wesorick B. Polarity thinking: an essential skill for those leading interprofessional integration. *J Interprof Healthcare.* 2014;1(1):1–17.

27. U.S. Institute of Medicine (IOM). *Redesigning Continuing Education in the Health Professions.* Washington, DC: The National Academies Press; 2010.

CHAPTER 9

Putting It All Together: The Age of Nursing and Allied Health Professionals

Like any good book, this last chapter is meant to bring it all together, to serve as a general summary of the many topics covered in the previous chapters, and to reiterate the key points and concepts, to help you successfully navigate as you travel along your healthcare provider journey. So, while right about now you may suddenly be wondering why you even bothered to read the previous chapters, I will modestly suggest that doing so wasn't a (complete) waste of your time, as there is (I hope) great value in having a deeper understanding of the major issues involved in the healthcare reform revolution.

And so to start off, this last chapter will first *begin at the beginning*.

No, not the beginning of time, nor even the beginning of the current healthcare reform revolution. Let's go back *to the beginning of this book*, to Chapter 1.

Our goal (as I shared way back then) was not simply for you to understand *the basics* of today's US healthcare reform. Rather, we sought to provide you with a *deeper understanding of both the drivers and the impact of reform to help you navigate your professional career through this actively changing healthcare environment.* And I was emphatic in stating that we need you to do more than simply successfully *navigate* healthcare reform. *We need you to lead* healthcare reform. I have argued throughout the book that *only if nurses and allied health professionals step up as leaders in reform will we truly have the opportunity to dramatically improve the health of our population and the value of our healthcare system.* I supported this argument (back in that first chapter) by reviewing the numbers:

- More than 325,000,000 patients and future patients are spread across the United States, a population that is aging
- The fact that there are only 442,000 primary care physicians and 484,000 specialist physicians (that's one primary care physician for every 735 Americans)[1]
- Physicians still overwhelmingly cluster around urban centers (geographic asymmetry), further reducing the physician-to-patient ratio in rural American regions (especially when it comes to access to specialty and sub-specialty physicians)[2]
- The enormous healthcare force is represented by the almost *3,200,000 registered nurses* and *827,000 licensed practical nurses* in the United States[3]
- *19.8 million allied health professionals* will be working in our healthcare system by 2020[4]

These numbers tell a story. A story of a large, aging population . Of limited physician availability. And of the significant army of nurses and allied health professionals available to step up and lead in improving the health of the American population and of the American healthcare system.

Next, we pointed out that the US Department of Labor (DOL) has publicly acknowledged the need for many, many more non-physicians to realize higher value health and healthcare, through the DOL's projected rankings of the "The Fastest Growing Occupations" from 2014 through 2024[5]:

#2—Occupational Therapy Assistants
#3—Physical Therapist Assistants
#4—Physical Therapist Aides
#5—Home Health Aides
#7—Nurse Practitioners
#8—Physical Therapists
#10—Ambulance Drivers and Attendants

I pointed out that *7 of the top 10 fastest growing occupations in the United States are non-physician healthcare providers or non-physician healthcare-related.* In fact, over the next decade, *20 of the 30 occupations projected to grow most rapidly are non-physician healthcare providers or non-physician healthcare-related,* including:

- Physician Assistants
- Genetic Counselors
- Audiologists
- Diagnostic Medical Sonographers
- Phlebotomists
- Nurse Midwives
- Emergency Medical Technicians
- Paramedics
- Optometrists

Thus, we began our educational journey together back in Chapter 1 by recognizing that *nurses and allied health professionals already comprise an enormous portion of our healthcare workforce,* and that *the number of these providers will continue to grow.* Thus, my final conclusion was clear:

Today's healthcare reform represents *The Age of Nursing and Allied Health Professionals.*

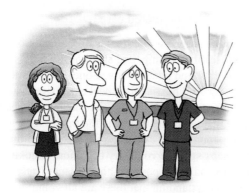

Next, to understand what it means today to practice in the midst of *The Perfect Healthcare Reform Storm,* we had to look back to where we (American healthcare) came from. You now appreciate that the traditional American healthcare reimbursement model is founded in one major concept: the dissociation between provider payment for care (reimbursement) from the quality of that delivered care. Within our American economy, this traditional *fee-for-service* care reimbursement system is a unique (but major economic) oddity, since it is the one large industry sector in which there lacks any relationship between value and payment. Thus, the sole Provider in this traditional fee-for-service model, the Doctor, is free from accountability for patient care outcomes that result from his or her professional services. Nor in the traditional American healthcare model do patients bear any meaningful responsibility for their own health and healthcare. Regardless of the behaviors, decisions, actions, and inactions, the healthcare system simply treated their poor health outcomes when they occurred and sent the patients back on their way. And we also discussed how nurses and allied health professionals are like patients in being relegated to passive roles in the traditional fee-for-service environment, expected to simply follow the physician's recommendations and instructions with little question or thought. Nurses, therapists, dieticians, technicians, and others are simply viewed (and referred to) as "physician extenders," of little value in the delivery of patient care in their own right.

> The traditional American healthcare reimbursement model is founded in one major concept: the dissociation between provider payment for care (reimbursement) from the quality of that delivered care.

So Doctors are the sole Captains of the Traditional American Healthcare Ship, and allied health professionals, nurses, patients, and patients' loved ones are the silent, obeying crew. And boy is this model expensive! The greatest cost comes from the passive role in both health and healthcare that the patients play in the traditional system plan. Long, long ago, we all accepted the proven links between many specific voluntary behaviors (smoking, over-eating) and many poor health outcomes (lung cancer, diabetes), understanding that these are all volun*tary behaviors which result in massive healthcare costs for us all* in hospitalizations, procedures, operations, medical treatments, ER visits, physical therapy, long-term care, etc., etc., etc. Adding to the enormous pile of wasted dollars are the fee-for-service-based physicians, who are rarely held accountable for their care outcomes (other than when sued for medical negligence), routinely practicing based solely on their training, experience, and intuition, feeling little pressure to keep current on "best practices." Thus, physicians spend money on diagnostic and therapeutic activities that offer little to no benefit. And that's just *unintentional*, unnecessary physician spending. The significant fear of malpractice lawsuits (particularly frivolous and questionable claims), and the absence of any penalty for over-ordering of tests and procedures, has ignited the *routine practice of defensive medicine*, wasting unbelievable mounds of *everyone's money* without benefitting patients. Is it any wonder that with unaccountable patients and unaccountable physicians practicing defensively that the healthcare reimbursement doled out by fee-for-service insurers and taxpayers (that is, *all of us*) has driven America to the brink of economic viability?

It is not.

But what is a wonder (and frustration, and source of great anger) is that for all of this over-the-top spending, the overall quality of our population's health and of traditional American healthcare is *terrible.* By any one of a number of rankings, US healthcare receives a failing grade (even when cost of care is not considered in the analysis).

This was and is our traditional American healthcare system. From not-too-great a distance, it was obvious that we were sailing directly into a massive storm in which multiple fronts were colliding, threatening to sink not only our healthcare system, but our entire economic ship . . .

> Is it any wonder that with unaccountable patients and unaccountable physicians practicing defensively that the healthcare reimbursement doled out by fee-for-service insurers and taxpayers (that is, *all of us*) has driven America to the brink of economic viability?

In the end (and perhaps not surprisingly), the healthcare reform revolution was not sparked by the poor overall quality of American healthcare. Nor was lack of a patient-centered focus or patient accountability the initiator of aggressive reform. Nor even the evidence demonstrating the value of interprofessional collaborative patient care. No, in the end, it was *the spiraling cost of US healthcare* that triggered alarms in the most influential political hallways. It was our *over-the-top healthcare spend accelerating towards 18% of our gross domestic product* that generated dire warnings from economists across the political spectrum. And in large part, while politicians, economists, and others began crying out for action, many clinicians simply buried our heads in the sand, hoping (many anticipating) that this most recent attempt at healthcare reform would pass like a brief storm, the way that previous reform efforts had passed.

But this time, *the storm did not pass.* Because unlike previous reform attempts, *this storm is a Level 5 hurricane.* This time, several powerful fronts have slammed into one another to form *The Perfect Healthcare Reform Storm.* Most critical was *the significant public awareness* of two threatening and opposing realities: the *unsustainable cost* of US healthcare and the *overwhelmingly poor clinical quality* of US healthcare. Add to this the lightning pace at which health and healthcare knowledge is exploding (in large part, as we rapidly unravel the riddles of genomics), and it became clear: this storm would not soon pass. This storm would, *must* permanently alter the American healthcare landscape.

And so here we are, in the midst of *The Perfect Healthcare Reform Storm,* with providers, patients, administrators, politicians, and other stakeholders all trying to navigate our way through to smoother waters. The politicians made the first move, and it was a doozy. They shattered the foundation of our traditional American healthcare system by *linking provider reimbursement with defined clinical outcomes.* And the most powerful aspect of that linkage is their "big stick:" heavily financially penalizing provider organizations for suboptimal clinical outcomes. As for the timeline of federally legislated reform, one certainly can argue that it is unrealistically aggressive (being based on political rather than operational realities in dramatically altering the complex system which contributes close to 18% of the gross domestic product). But to argue that we should not move away from fee-to-service to a value-based care model, *a healthcare system in which there is a relationship between the value of delivered care (quality and cost) with payment,* is a thin argument indeed. Such value-based care represents a critical pivot away from low quality, high cost healthcare; that is, value-based care points our ship in the right direction, aiming us toward the safest course through the storm and on to a healthier (and more financially stable) nation.

> The politicians made the first move, and it was a doozy. They shattered the foundation of our traditional American healthcare system by *linking provider reimbursement with defined clinical outcomes.*

And while no, the ACA ("ObamaCare") is far from perfect, no one should have expected this major attempt at meaningful reform to be perfect. As other nations' experiences are now confirming, it is *entirely unrealistic to expect that we will "get it right the first time"* when trying to radically alter a complex, multi-tiered healthcare system that impacts every one of us (as patients and/ or payers). The revolution driving us towards better population health and high value healthcare will, in fact, mimic an actual military revolution. Victory will not be realized after the first battle, even if that initial assault is significant. Rather, this revolution will be won only after years of battles and skirmishes with healthcare leaders analyzing successes and failures and then subsequently implementing modified actions in our march towards victory.

What the Healthcare Reform Revolution Means for You

So, what does this healthcare reform revolution mean for nurses and allied health professionals in general, and for you specifically?

Simply said, today's American healthcare reform revolution represents *the greatest professional opportunity for non-physician providers in American healthcare history.*

Think of it. We are now sailing towards multiple, bold, complementary goals:

- *Cost-efficient healthcare that is consistently of high quality and is embedded in one or more sustainable models*
- *A significantly healthier nation*
- *Dramatically increased "health ownership" by patients*
- *A shift from reactive, acute, in-hospital care to proactive, out-of-hospital, preventive, and maintenance care*

And it will be, *it must be nurses and allied health professionals who lead us on this journey.* Not based solely on the numbers we have just reviewed, but more importantly, because *no other providers (physicians included) spend as much time and develop such broad and deep relationships with patients* and their loved ones as do nurses and allied health professionals. Indeed, *practicing at the top of your license demands gaining a meaningful understanding of your patients.* Thus, allied health professionals and nurses are primed to play the major role in driving towards these bold, complementary healthcare reform goals.

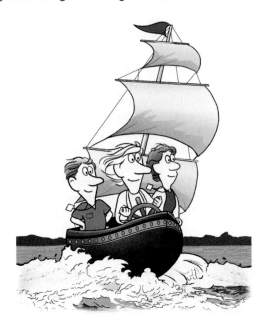

But this tremendous responsibility *should not be viewed as a burden.* Rather, *it is an amazing opportunity!* No longer are you "physician extenders," nameless assistants standing behind doctors, perceived as of minimal individual value in the patient care process. You are now truly *critical* PROVIDERS. You now play key roles in achieving value-based care, in advancing Population Health Management, in driving impactful Patient Engagement, Patient Education, and Patient Empowerment. You, nurses and allied health professionals, you will be leading us towards proactive, out-of-hospital, preventive and maintenance care. You will be empowering our population to improve their health and their lives. And you will be foundational in transforming the world of healthcare into one in which patients consistently receive the highest quality care, and all of us pay only what is necessary to provide that highest quality care.

And Our Educational Institutions?

Yes, the day of the Doctor as THE PROVIDER is over. But successful healthcare reform demands more than just expanding our PROVIDER list. Just by recognizing the value of radiology technicians, medical assistants, speech therapists, other allied health professionals, and nurses as essential providers is not enough to reach our laudable reform goals. Consistent, sustainable value-based care demands that individual provider types *no longer function in isolation,* each focusing only on "their area" of patient care. No, consistent, sustainable, high value healthcare *demands teamwork.* Only when collaborative, interprofessional care *becomes the norm,* the accepted and expected model for the provision of patient care, will our society take a major step towards consistent, sustainable, high-value healthcare. Nor can we teach such a team approach, in which providers truly understand and appreciate one another's scopes-of-practice, in which providers feel comfortable in openly communicating with one another about any and all aspects of patient care, only once our student-providers have graduated; that is, we can't first introduce interprofessional collaborative care in our actual patient care settings. No, *interprofessional collaborative care must first be introduced in the classroom.* Our nursing students, respiratory therapy students, occupational therapy students, radiology technician students, dieticians-in-training, other allied health professional students and, yes, medical students *must be educated within an interprofessional care framework.* Future providers must matriculate *already viewing interprofessional collaborative care as normal* as hand washing between patient exams. As simply as *how the best healthcare is delivered.*

This sounds easier than it is (and it doesn't even sound that easy). Because successfully educating students in various disciplines to think interprofessionally from the get-go requires educators who both believe and are well versed in interprofessional education and collaborative practice (IPECP). And there is a paucity of healthcare professional educators experienced in practicing (let alone teaching) IPECP. Still, we're only just beginning, and as with all such "flip-the-system-on-its-head" movements, things will improve quickly with further experience.

And the Ultimate Providers?

As I've said, true population health improvement and healthcare reform will only be fully realized *when patients seize ownership of their behaviors, decisions, and health.* But it will take a great deal of time and commitment to turn our society into one in which individuals "own their health." As with the government's preferred "big stick" for "encouraging" provider organizations to improve the value of delivered care, significant financial penalties may ultimately be the prod utilized by the government (and/or private insurers) to "encourage" individual Americans to make healthier lifestyle choices. Whether up front (an extreme example: taxation based on body mass index) or after entering the healthcare system (an extreme example: once a smoker's insurance reaches a cap, they can no longer receive treatment for their lung cancer), if healthcare spending doesn't clearly slow in a meaningful way as a result of penalties levied against *providers* (and it may not, particularly in the absence of tort reform to rein in medical malpractice lawsuits), individual Americans may find themselves targeted for painful financial penalizations based on their health and healthcare decisions.

And so, until patients themselves begin to truly accept accountability and responsibility for their personal health and healthcare decisions, we trained healthcare professionals must guide those patients (and our society as a whole) through the storm. But *we must trumpet the goal of having our patients step up into the role of the ultimate PROVIDER.*

> We trained healthcare professionals *must trumpet the goal of having our patients step up into the role of the ultimate PROVIDER.*

For some providers, this change to patient-centered health ownership may be difficult to accept (let alone encourage), as it means abandoning our traditional place atop America's healthcare pedestal and our historic responsibility as the owners of our patients' healthcare decisions. Especially if you're an older provider (like this physician), the patient-centric and patient ownership concepts so critical to the successful reform represent a dynamic shift in how we providers will be perceived by society and perhaps even in how we perceive ourselves. We will move from "leaders" to "partners." But this is evolution in the positive sense, moving us as a whole towards a healthier society (as well as a more economically stable one). And I encourage you to consider something else: *your career satisfaction may actually increase* by embracing this patient-as-the-ultimate-PROVIDER concept. By partnering with patients and their loved ones to achieve greater health, to prevent illness, to avoid emergency room visits, and *to reduce preventable pain and suffering and death,* you will truly advance yourself as a healthcare provider. You will be helping your patients and your society in achieving something that has never before been achieved: a healthier, happier, more economically stable America.

> *Your career satisfaction may actually increase* by embracing this patient-as-the-ultimate-PROVIDER concept.

With consistent, aggressive provider encouragement (and potentially with legislated carrots and sticks), patients will eventually accept at least increased health ownership. Hopefully we will reach critical mass sooner rather than later, as individual health ownership is a key to the realization of a healthier nation and consistent, high value healthcare.

> Individual health ownership is a key to the realization of a healthier nation and consistent, high value healthcare.

Broken down into its major components, health ownership is comprised of three sequential phases that must be continuously reinforced: Patient Engagement, (then) Patient Education, and (finally) Patient Empowerment. And once again, nurses and allied health professionals are the providers in the optimal position to drive this challenging-yet-critical process. Certainly, physicians are important as well in driving patient health ownership, but the nature of the interactions and relationships forged between patients and families with non-physician providers offer the best chance to change our society's perception of health ownership.

As I've said, *the key is partnership.* And also work to partner with your patient's loved ones, including family, friends, clergy, and all who demonstrate a personal investment in your patient. *Repeatedly* encourage (even strongly) the benefits of and need for your patients to own their health *based on what you've learned of them as individuals.* Be the provider partner who truly gets to know and appreciates their values, goals, dreams, and fears, as this will empower you to help them truly engage in their own health. And once engaged, patients and their loved ones are open to become educated and, ultimately, empowered. Be your patients' *clinical partner and advocate,* and you will see their health improve, healthcare needs and costs lessen, and your own professional satisfaction grow.

> Be your patients' *clinical partner and advocate,* and you will see their health improve, healthcare needs and costs lessen, and your own professional satisfaction grow.

And Population Health Management?

The pathway to successful population health management (PHM) mimics that leading to successful patient engagement. Again, physicians play a key role in helping define target populations for interventions and education (based on clinical characteristics and identified risks), but true population health management requires much more than simply stratifying patients by disease or condition and then providing purely clinical interventions to reduce or eliminate health risks. Focusing solely through a clinical lens will significantly limit the success of any PHM program. To realize maximal success, we cannot only provide glucose monitoring instructions to a population of poorly controlled, elderly type 2 diabetics. We can't just give bathroom scales to a group of struggling heart failure patients. PHM requires that *we understand our patients as more than just diseases and conditions.* That we break these groups down into individuals, understand their personal values, family resources, financial stresses, literacy and language challenges. In the end, it may well turn out that there are more successful ways to divide groups but better understanding their nonclinical issues as well. Why are these diabetics and heart failure patients struggling? Perhaps a better "population" for management will be some of the diabetics and some of the heart failure patients who share a common problem: a language or transportation or support system challenge. It is in this recognition, in *seeing the management of a population's health and the engagement of the individuals within that population as bookends,* that lays the path to improved societal health and consistent, high value healthcare. And as such, PHM (like patient engagement) requires the development of personal relationships with individuals within the larger populations (especially those identified as most likely to benefit from such interactions). Such relationship building takes time, commitment, and compassion along with an understanding of the clinical scenario. That is why nurses, therapists, dieticians, medical assistants, and many other allied health professionals are in the best position to lead our PHM efforts.

Don't Get Overwhelmed!

So, let's review. Nurses and allied health professionals *must dramatically expand their clinical knowledge and patient care skills,* as healthcare reform is demanding both broader and deeper care to be provided by these non-physician providers. *Check.*

Allied health professionals and nurses must play leading roles in driving consistent, sustainable, high quality, cost-efficient healthcare. That is, these allied health professionals *must practice value-based care. Got it.*

Nurses and allied health professionals *must drive Patient Engagement, Patient Education, and Patient Empowerment,* as attaining an increased level of patient health ownership is critical in improving the health of our society. *OK.*

Same thing for Population Health Management. Allied health professionals and nurses *must provide leadership* for this component of the Triple Aim to be achieved. *Fair enough.*

And *interprofessional education and collaborative care must be advanced* through the leadership of nurse and allied health professionals for the benefits of meaningful healthcare reform to be realized. *Understood.*

Ready to quit?

Don't! Remember, *all of these new demands on you and your colleagues represent wonderful opportunities* for you to play critical roles in improving the health and healthcare of your patients and of the entire American society. Opportunities for *you. You.*

There are so many roads down which you can travel today (and tomorrow). So much you can learn, so many new skills you can acquire, so many new ways to benefit your patients and increase your own professional satisfaction. Clinical knowledge, procedural skills, administrative experience, interprofessional care and education, etc., etc. Opportunities unknown to all but a few of the nurses and allied health professionals who practiced before this moment in healthcare history. So *seize the opportunity, accept the challenge, provide even broader and deeper direct patient care,* and *find even greater professional satisfaction* as you step up to the front in the greatest single effort to improve the health and healthcare in our country's history.

But *you can't truly succeed without help.* And here I'm not talking about the help and guidance of other providers (which you certainly should seek out and offer throughout your career). I'm talking about the help you will need from the moment you enter training to the moment you place down your stethoscope or other instrument-of-choice for the last time. The help that is now demanded by value-based care to keep current with the massive health and healthcare knowledge explosion. To always know what represents the "best practice" in the care of your patients. Because today, you must provide the highest quality of clinical care by *only doing all of the right things, only doing them in the right order, only doing them at the right time, and never doing anything unnecessary, or in the wrong order, or at the wrong time.* And you must *absolutely, positively avoid preventable medical errors that lead to patient injuries and patient deaths.*

You can't truly succeed without help. I'm talking about the help you will need from the moment you enter training to the moment you place down your stethoscope or other instrument-of-choice for the last time. The help that is now demanded by value-based care to keep current with the massive health and healthcare knowledge explosion.

For those of you who have worked in the business world, these are known as "stretch goals." Stretch goals are bold, audacious, and nearly impossible to achieve. And yet for endeavors as important and universal as those set for our society by healthcare reform, stretch goals are inspiring, as they represent "goals for ourselves that uplift the human spirit, goals that inspire those doing work and delight those for whom work is done[6]." Will we ever achieve a zero rate for preventable medical errors? Extremely unlikely, given the reliance of health and healthcare safety on human actions (providers and patients). But it is a laudable goal. An appropriate goal for which we should as providers and patients and taxpayers and members of a society should strive for. Should *stretch* for. And it is one of the stretch goals which you as an individual provider and member of a patient care team should stretch for, always, and encourage others (including your patients) to stretch for.

The struggle to advance toward your (and our) stretch goals demands current, credible, evidence-based information at our fingertips. Even if our species never learned a single thing more about the human body, physiology, disease, medications, surgical treatments…there will still already be way, way too much care knowledge for any one provider to remember, let alone master (even in a narrowly focused practice). And the reality is far (far!) from this hypothetical. The genomics explosion has driven our scientific knowledge to accelerate at a pace never seen before in the history of human research and discovery. Everything humans know about health and healthcare will soon double every 2 months. New diagnostic tests. New medications. Gene modification treatments! Nor can we continue to ignore nonclinical patient issues, such as patient socio-demographics, patient finances, patient support systems, patient values and wishes…

There is simply so much to know, on which to stay current, to take into account. Overwhelming. With so much to know, to consider, *how will you keep up?*

Enter *Clinical Decision Support.* These solutions (whether in print or integrated into an electronic health record) are already available to support nurses, physicians, patients, pharmacists, and a variety of allied health professionals. Clinical decision support (CDS) solutions provide *rapid access to current, credible, evidence-based information, the foundation of value-based care.* And not only are provider discipline-specific CDS solutions growing in number, *interprofessional CDS solutions* (such as care plans and clinical pathways) are already available, with additional collaborative team solutions soon to hit the market.

> Clinical decision support solutions provide *rapid access to current, credible, evidence-based information, the foundation of value-based care.*

For many of us older providers, the thought of having to learn to navigate through a variety of new technological solutions and gadgets while still meeting our overly busy clinical demands fills us with angst. I have no magic bullet here, only some suggestions. First of all, *volunteer whenever there is an opportunity to participate in your organization's evaluation of health information technology (HIT) solutions.* While this will cost you time up front, by doing so, you can influence your organization's technology purchases, factoring in ease-of-use, integration into other solutions, and other characteristics that truly matter to providers based on your own knowledge and work experience. And before casting your vote to purchase an HIT solution, require the vendor to arrange for you to visit a facility where that specific CDS solution is being used by providers like you. Speak to those providers or, better yet, visit them and see the HIT tool in action. Second, as part of the purchase agreement, *require that the selected vendor provide on-site support* in the wards and units over a specified period of initial solution implementation (for very complex solutions in high volume organizations, that vendor support might even need to be 24/7 for several weeks). In this way, those less tech-savvy providers will feel less stressed and will more quickly learn (through vendor-supported use) how to integrate the newly purchased HIT product into their workflow. Finally, *ask other provider types for their input* even if the solution you're evaluating is designed for use by one specific provider type. For example, if you're evaluating a CDS solution for physical therapists, ask nurses, physicians, and other providers who also routinely care for those patients for their thoughts on the product under evaluation.

And remember this: *technology itself (such as an electronic health record) is limited in its innate ability to empower the delivery of high value care. Information is the massive force which drives consistent, sustainable, high value care.* And accessing the right information in the right location at the right time is the most powerful way to ensure that your patients receive care of the highest quality while we all (you, me, insurers) pay no more than necessary.

> And remember this: *technology itself (such as an electronic health record) is limited in its innate ability to empower the delivery of high value care. Information is the massive force which drives consistent, sustainable, high value care.*

Thus, your information must come from a *credible source* (and remember, *credible* information is rarely free). Your information must always *remain current* (another reason that the best patient care information costs money). And the highest value information is *evidence-based.* It should be available on mobile devices. It should draw from current, credible, evidence-based resources which are appropriate in format and style for the provider types using the solution (as different disciplines understand and adopt information differently). It must provide rapid answers to your questions, and better yet, *it should provide answers to knowledge gaps that you are unaware you have* (CDS push solutions)! It must be intuitive and easy to use. It must interrupt your workflow to as minimal an extent as possible.

And you must work hard to incorporate these powerful information solutions into your workflow. Yes, it is true that integrating new technology into your busy workflow frequently slows you down, reduces your efficiency, stresses and frustrates you. *Initially.* But like any new technology, in time (often in short order), you'll grow comfortable with both the technology and the place of that technology within your daily workflow. (Remember when you bought your first smartphone? It didn't take long to master it, and now it's never far from your hand!)

Now Is Your Time

Yes, we are in the midst of *The Perfect Healthcare Reform Storm.* But for the nurse and for the allied health professional who understands the forces that have created this storm, who has the right bearing and is navigating directly towards smooth waters and clear skies, today's health reform represents something other than a storm. It represents *The Age of Nursing and Allied Health Professionals.*

So get out there and lead our patients and our society to better health, our healthcare system to economic sustainability, and yourself to a tremendously satisfying career.

References

1. The Henry J. Kaiser Family Foundation. 2016. (online) http://kff.org/other/state-indicator/total-active-physicians/?currentTimeframe=0.
2. Rosenthal MB, Zaslavsky A, Newhouse JP. The geographic distribution of physicians revisited. *Health Serv Res.* 2005;40:1931–1952.
3. The Henry J. Kaiser Family Foundation. 2016. (online) http://kff.org/other/state-indicator/total-registered-nurses/?currentTimeframe=0.
4. The Association of Schools of Allied Health Professions (ASAHP). (online) http://www.asahp.org/wp-content/uploads/2014/08/Health-Professions-Facts.pdf.
5. U.S. Department of Labor, Bureau of Labor Statistics. 2014–2024 projections. (online) https://www.bls.gov/emp/ep_table_103.htm.
6. Denning S. In Praise of Stretch Goals. *Forbes* (online). 2012. https://www.forbes.com/sites/stevedenning/2012/04/23/in-praise-of-stretch-goals/#4e63995b7c04.

CHAPTER 10

Simple Glossary of Healthcare Reform Terms and Abbreviations

Throughout this book, you will find words and terms in **bold print.** These words and terms are more extensively defined and explained here in this Glossary of Terms. Note that many healthcare terms (particularly those associated with today's healthcare reform) often have more than one (even multiple) definitions, as uniform agreement has not yet been reached (for example, "evidence-based practice"). In other cases, many people use two similar terms interchangeably, even though additional study demonstrates that subtle differences exist between the terms (e.g., "electronic *medical* record" and "electronic *health* record"). Where multiple definitions or uses of a term are common, I have done my best to provide you with the definition or concept consistent with the points being made in this work. In many cases, I directly quote and cite a source whose definition and explanation is consistent with that used in this book.

Affordable Care Act (ACA) The *Patient Protection and Affordable Care Act* (the *ACA*, also referred to as "*The Affordable Care Act*" and "*ObamaCare*") was signed into federal law in 2010. The primary stated goal of the ACA is to *dramatically increase access to affordable healthcare coverage.* The ACA has additional goals, such as reducing wasteful spending, expanding Medicaid, and improving the quality of healthcare and of Americans' health (to name only a few).[1]

Accountable Care Organizations (ACOs) "Accountable Care Organizations (ACOs) are groups of doctors, hospitals, and other healthcare providers, who come together voluntarily to give coordinated high quality care to the Medicare patients they serve. Coordinated care helps ensure that patients, especially the chronically ill, get the right care at the right time, with the goal of avoiding unnecessary duplication of services and preventing medical errors."[2] ACOs can share in financial savings if they achieve government-specified quality outcomes at reduced costs (few ACOs have realized significant shared savings at the time of this writing). However, ACOs can also be financially penalized for failing to deliver government-specified quality, cost-efficient care.

Care Plans Care Plans come in a variety of forms. Overall, the goal of a Care Plan is to delineate the steps in assessment (and reassessment) and care of an individual patient across care settings. Most Care Plans also guide providers in the creation of patient-specific problem lists, offering information on patient-specific goals and guidance to address the identified problems as care moves forward. While frequently perceived as specifically (or only) for use by nurses, Care Plans are now available for use by multiple provider disciplines and even by interprofessional teams, allowing for collaborative patient care.

Centers for Disease Control and Prevention (CDC) Within the US Department of Health and Human Services, "The Centers for Disease Control and Prevention (CDC) serves as the national focus for developing and applying disease prevention and control, environmental health, and health promotion and health education activities designed to improve the health of the people of the United States."[3]

Clinical Decision Support (CDS) "Clinical decision support (CDS) provides timely information, usually at the point of care, to help inform decisions about a patient's care. CDS tools and systems help clinical teams by taking over some routine tasks, warning of potential problems, or providing suggestions for the clinical team and patient to consider. The main purpose of CDS is to provide timely information to clinicians, patients, and others to inform decisions about health care."[4] Through the pushing and pulling of current, credible, evidence-based information and guidance, CDS solutions are among our most powerful tools in achieving consistent, sustainable, high quality, cost-efficient healthcare.

CPOE Initially the acronym for *Computerized Physician Order Entry* (given that physicians enter the overwhelming majority of patient orders), the term has been expanded to mean *Computerized Provider Order Entry.* "CPOE entails the provider's use of computer assistance to directly enter medication orders from a computer or mobile device. The order is also documented or captured in a digital, structured, and computable format for use in improving safety and organization."[5]

Defensive Medicine "Medical practices designed to avert the future possibility of malpractice suits. In defensive medicine, responses are undertaken primarily to avoid liability rather than to benefit the patient. Doctors [and other providers] may order tests, procedures, or visits, or avoid high-risk patients or procedures primarily (but not necessarily solely) to reduce their exposure to malpractice liability."[6] The practice of defensive medicine by individual providers and provider organizations is widely perceived as a major driver of unnecessary testing and procedures and, thus, as a leading cause of significant, unnecessary healthcare spending.

Evidence-Based Wow, are there a lot of "evidence-based" terms and definitions! At its narrowest, "evidence-based research" and "evidence-based medicine" are the processes of using basic (bench) and clinical scientific research, respectively (such as rigorously designed clinical trials) to determine the best scientific approaches to the diagnosis, treatment, and prevention of diseases and conditions. The term "evidence-based practice" is significantly broader and is gaining popularity. This term usually implies the inclusion of evidence-based research and evidence-based medicine but adds to this information gleaned from provider experience and, importantly, patient values, culture, and input.[7] To many, evidence-based practice favorably adds "the art of medicine" and "the human element" to the concept of evidence-based care.

Evidence-Informed "Some people use the terms evidence-based and evidence-informed interchangeably … However, evidence-informed is … the 'catchphrase' of choice as it appears to provide more flexibility regarding the nature of the evidence and its use, i.e., it implies that many different levels of evidence and types of evidence

[such as qualitative studies and 'common sense']
are needed and used to support decisions in clinical
practice."[8] As in the case of "evidence-based medicine"
versus "evidence-based practice," many supporters favor
the inclusion of "the art of medicine" and "the human
element" represented by the "evidence-informed" practice
concept.

Electronic Health Record (EHR) "An electronic health
record (EHR) is a digital version of a patient's paper
chart. EHRs are real-time, patient-centered records that
make information available instantly and securely to
authorized users. While an EHR does contain the medical
and treatment histories of patients [including out-of-
hospital care], an EHR system is built to go beyond
standard clinical data collected in a provider's office and
can be inclusive of a broader view of a patient's care
[including information on the patient's socio-demographic
characteristics, support network, spirituality, etc.]."[9] The
term "EHR" is rapidly replacing the older term, "electronic
medical record (EMR)," which refers to a digital record
of a hospitalized patient and is more narrowly focused on
purely clinical (medical and surgical) care issues.[10]

Fee-for-Service Although there are several variations,
fee-for-service is a reimbursement model in which the
physician, other providers, and provider organizations
receive payment for each service (test, procedure, patient
evaluation, etc.) performed. At its core, *fee-for-service
financially rewards providers for volume of services* (that
is, the model pays providers more for doing more) and
*has no meaningful connection between payment to the
provider and the quality or cost-efficiency of the care
delivered by the provider.* Fee-for-service is the basic
reimbursement model of the traditional (pre-reform)
American healthcare system.

Frivolous Malpractice Lawsuit Frivolous malpractice
lawsuits are legal claims of negligent, damaging care
that in reality do not meet the required legal standards.
In lay terms, these are patient (or patient family) lawsuits
that lack any merit, often viewed as driven by unethical
malpractice attorneys and/or clients seeking to make
money off of providers when no negligence actually
occurred and/or the patient did not suffer any meaningful
harm. It is estimated that "about 40 percent of the medical
malpractice cases filed in the United States are groundless
[frivolous]."[11] Frivolous lawsuits significantly drive up the
costs of healthcare for all of us, not only from the payment
of lawsuit settlements (which some insurers prefer to the

costs of fighting a frivolous suit in court), but most gravely by triggering the widespread, costly (and, for patients, nonbeneficial) practice of defensive medicine. The absence of tort reform (modification of the medical malpractice litigation laws) in the Affordable Care Act is considered by many a significant flaw which limits the legislation's ability to reduce unnecessary care costs.

Genomics (the human genome; our DNA) "DNA is the chemical compound that contains the instructions needed to develop and direct the activities of nearly all living organisms. ... An organism's [including a human's] complete set of DNA is called its genome."[12] Everything about you (hair color, likelihood of cancer, intelligence, height, personality quirks) is completely or heavily influenced by the "blueprint of you," the DNA found in your cells; that is, your personal genome. The study of the human genome (such as searching for the relationship between DNA mistakes, called "mutations," and diseases) is called "genomics." The recent explosion in our understanding of genomics represents the greatest and most rapid advance in the history of health and healthcare, and the healthcare of the near future will likely bear little resemblance to that of yesterday, as genomics discoveries are changing disease prevention and treatment in ways only previously dreamed of in *Star Trek* and other science fiction worlds.

Gross Domestic Product (GDP) GDP is a measurement of "the value of the goods and services produced by the U.S. economy in a given time period"[13] (including the salaries of the workers who produce those goods and services[14]). As such, GDP is among the most frequently utilized, cited, and critically followed economic indicators for the United States and other nations. At the time of this writing, spending on healthcare in the United States exceeds 17% of America's GDP, widely seen as economically non-viable.

Health Information Technology (HIT) Health information technology "is a broad concept that encompasses an array of technologies to store, share, and analyze health information. More and more, healthcare providers are using health IT to improve patient care. ... [In addition, patients] can use health IT to better communicate with ... doctor[s], learn and share information about ... [their] health, and take actions that will improve [their] quality of life."[15] The hope is that "Widespread use of health IT within the health care industry will improve the quality of health care, prevent medical errors, reduce health care costs, increase administrative efficiencies, decrease paperwork, and expand access to affordable health care."[16] Electronic health records and many clinical decision support solutions are examples of HIT.

Health Literacy "Health literacy is the degree to which individuals have the capacity to obtain, process and understand basic health information needed to make appropriate health decisions."[17] The term is generally thought of as referring to a patient's ability to understand the written and spoken word (care instructions, explanations of tests and procedures, etc.).

Health Numeracy Sometimes lumped together under "Health Literacy," health numeracy refers to a patient's ability to understand numerical aspects of care (medication dosage, medication frequency, risk statistics, disease incidence and prevalence, etc.).

Healthcare Reimbursement Model "Reimbursement" simply means payment, and in the healthcare setting refers to payments made by patients, private insurers, taxpayers (via Medicare, Medicaid, and similar government-sponsored programs) to individual providers, provider groups, and provider organizations. A "model" describes the structure of payment. For example, *fee-for-service* and *value-based reimbursement* are two models; the former dissociates reimbursement and patient care metrics, while the latter has a significant relationship between reimbursement and defined care value.

Healthcare Value While there are numerous definitions of "value" floating around today, in its simplest form, "healthcare value" equals the quality of care divided by the cost of care. Stated differently, higher quality care and/or lower cost care results in greater healthcare value.

HIMSS The *Healthcare Information and Management Systems Society* describes itself as "a global, cause-based, not-for-profit organization focused on better health through information technology (IT)."[18] Across the world, HIMSS is widely viewed as the accepted creator of the standards defining levels of health information technology (HIT) capabilities for use in advancing patient care.

HITECH Act "The Health Information Technology for Economic and Clinical Health (HITECH) Act of 2009 provides HHS [U.S. Department of Health and Human Services] with the authority to establish programs to improve health care quality, safety, and efficiency through the promotion of health IT, including electronic health records and private and secure electronic health information exchange."[19] In preceding the ACA, the HITECH Act laid the groundwork for the use of HIT as a critical foundational component of healthcare reform.

Hospital Consumer Assessment of Healthcare Providers and Systems (HCAHPS) "The intent of the HCAHPS initiative is to provide a standardized survey instrument and data collection methodology for measuring patients' perspectives on hospital care. … In order to make 'apples to apples' comparisons to support consumer choice, it was necessary to introduce a standard measurement approach."[20] Federal legislation requires that the "HCAHPS survey is administered to a random sample of adult patients across medical conditions between 48 hours and six weeks after discharge … Hospitals must survey patients throughout each month of the year. The Patient Protection and Affordable Care Act of 2010 [ACA] includes HCAHPS among the measures to be used to calculate value-based incentive payments [that is, HCCHPS scores are used in calculating Medicare reimbursement to provider organizations, addressing the 'Patient Experience' aim of the Triple Aim]."[21]

Institute for Healthcare Improvement (IHI) Considered across the globe as a premier healthcare think-tank, the Institute for Healthcare Improvement is "an independent not-for-profit organization … a leading innovator, convener, partner, and driver of results in health and health care improvement worldwide. … [The IHI has] partnered with visionaries, leaders, and front-line practitioners around the globe to spark bold, inventive ways to improve the health of individuals and populations."[22] IHI reports serve as major drivers of healthcare legislation and practice, and the release of major new IHI reports is often widely reported in both the industry and lay media.

Integrated Delivery Network (IDN) "An Integrated Delivery Network is a formal system of providers and sites of care that provides both health care services and a health insurance plan to patients in a particular geographic area. The functionalities … vary but can include acute care, long-term health, specialty clinics, primary care, and home care services, all supporting an owned health plan. To be a true IDN, a health system must offer a full set of complementary services; in contrast to other health systems which can serve as a collection of hospitals with similar capabilities."[23] To address the financial challenges posed by healthcare reform, many hospitals and hospital networks are expanding their services, developing into IDNs, providing them with greater control over health plan costs by influencing care delivery in both the inpatient and ambulatory care settings.

Interprofessional Care While definitions vary, they are routinely consistent with this definition: "Care delivered by intentionally created, usually relatively small work groups in health care, who are recognized by others as well as by themselves as having a collective identity and shared responsibility for a patient or group of patients, e.g., rapid response team, palliative care team, primary care team, operating room team." [24] As the term implies, interprofessional care involves patient care delivery by providers representing more than one discipline. While it is true that in the traditional American healthcare system, patient care involves multiple provider types, "interprofessional care" implies at least *coordinated* (and preferably *collaborative*) care among and across the differing providers and provider types, a significant difference from the traditional care model.

Interprofessional Education (IPE) IPE occurs when provider students from differing disciplines are educated (at least in part) together and when the overall educational focus for all provider-type students is on interprofessional care, collaborative practice, and patient-centered healthcare delivery.

Interprofessional Education and Collaborative Practice (IPECP) The full spectrum concept, starting with the interprofessional education (IPE) of student-providers from differing disciplines and leading to the collaborative practice (CP) of patient-centered, evidence-based care delivered by a functional team of providers from differing disciplines.

Malpractice Litigation The process of filing a civil lawsuit (legal claim) against one or more providers and/or provider organizations based on allegations of medically negligent care delivery resulting in harm (injury) to the plaintiff (usually the patient or patient's family). In the United States, medical malpractice laws are created and enforced on a state (rather than a federal) level.[25] Malpractice lawsuits (particularly frivolous suits) are widely viewed as playing a major role in the high cost of American healthcare.

Meaningful Use "Meaningful use ... [utilizes] certified electronic health record (EHR) technology to:

- Improve quality, safety, efficiency, and reduce health disparities
- Engage patients and family

- Improve care coordination, and population and public health
- Maintain privacy and security of patient health information

Ultimately, it is hoped that the meaningful use compliance will result in:

- Better clinical outcomes
- Improved population health outcomes
- Increased transparency and efficiency
- Empowered individuals
- More robust research data on health systems

Meaningful use sets specific objectives that eligible professionals (EPs) and hospitals must achieve to qualify for Centers for Medicare & Medicaid Services (CMS) Incentive Programs."[26] In basic terms, meaningful use is the federally mandated use of EHR technology capabilities at advancing levels to receive Medicare reimbursement and avoid financial penalization.

Medicaid "Medicaid provides health coverage to millions of Americans, including eligible low-income adults, children, pregnant women, elderly adults and people with disabilities. Medicaid is administered by states, according to federal requirements. The program is funded jointly by states and the federal government."[27] And in reality, *Medicaid is funded by you and me;* that is, by taxpayers. Thus, waste in the Medicaid system wastes our tax money.

Medicare "Medicare is the federal health insurance program for people age 65 or older, under 65 with certain disabilities, and any age with end-stage renal disease (permanent kidney failure requiring dialysis or a kidney transplant).
Medicare has four parts:

- Part A is hospital insurance.
- Part B is medical insurance.
- Part C Medical Advantage Plans are a private insurance option for covering hospital and medical costs.
- Part D covers prescription medications."[28]

And the truth is that *Medicare is funded by you and me;* that is, by taxpayers. Thus, waste in the Medicare system wastes our tax money.

ObamaCare The name often used in the lay press and in public referring to *The Patient Protection and Affordable Care Act* (the ACA, which was signed into law in 2010).

Office of the National Coordinator for Health Information Technology (ONC) "ONC is the principal federal entity charged with coordination of nationwide efforts to implement and use the most advanced health information technology and the electronic exchange of health information." Created in 2004 through a Presidential Executive Order, the ONC was legislated in 2009 through the HITECH Act to sit "at the forefront of the administration's health IT efforts and is a resource to the entire health system to support the adoption of health information technology and the promotion of nationwide health information exchange to improve health care."[29]

Outpatient and Ambulatory Surgery Consumer Assessment of Healthcare Providers and Systems (OAS CAHPS) This outpatient survey "collects information about patients' experiences of care in hospital outpatient departments (HOPDs) and ambulatory surgery centers (ASCs). … Considering the growing number of ASCs and the increase in Medicare expenditures for outpatient surgical services in both ASCs and HOPDs, the implementation of OAS CAHPS will provide statistically valid data from the patient perspective to inform quality improvement and comparative consumer information about outpatient facilities."[30] The ambulatory equivalent of the inpatient (HCAHPS) survey, the OAS CAHPS evaluates the ambulatory patient's "experience of care" and will play a role in determining Medicare provider reimbursement as part of the ASC Quality Reporting Program beginning in 2018.[31]

Patient Engagement Driving individual patients and their loved ones to truly accept accountability and responsibility in their own health and healthcare decisions and behaviors is an enormously challenging, complicated, and chronic process. Healthcare reform demands the significant engagement of patients, after which Patient Education (targeted to the individual patient's specific clinical scenario and non-clinical characteristics and values) and Patient Empowerment can occur. There are many reasons (often simultaneous) which lead patients to remain disengaged from their health issues and activities, including language and cultural challenges, as well as psychological dissociation of choices and outcomes. Thus, the process of patient engagement requires human and financial resources, expertise, and appropriate time allocation. While engagement of large portions of our population will take commitment and time, success is required to meaningfully improve America's health and healthcare.

Patient Experience of Care This is one of the three stated goals of the Triple Aim, the high-level roadmap for healthcare reform created by the Institute for Health Information and adopted by the US government. This aim component represents the first time that there is a mandated (via reimbursement penalties) national focus on both the patient's perceived quality of care and the patient's satisfaction with their overall care experience. Through the use of HCAHPS (and soon, OAS CAHPS), the patient experience (including several non-clinical aspects of the patient's interaction with the healthcare system) are evaluated and utilized for reimbursement decisions.[32]

Patient-Centered Care A foundational tenet of current healthcare reform, this model of care moves us away from the traditional focus on the physician and on the patient's disease to a view of health and healthcare in which "patients become active participants in their own care and receive services designed to focus on their individual needs and preferences, in addition to advice and counsel from health professionals."[33] Thus, patient-centered care is heavily influenced by the level of patient engagement and by the commitment of providers to partner with (rather than direct) patients in care decisions.

Patient-Centered Medical Home The Patient-Centered Medical Home is a care delivery model aimed at improving healthcare value "by transforming how primary care is organized and delivered. ... [and] encompasses five functions and attributes:

1. *Comprehensive Care:* ... accountable for meeting the large majority of each patient's physical and mental health care needs, including prevention and wellness, acute care, and chronic care ...
2. *Patient-Centered:* ... provides health care that is relationship-based with an orientation toward the whole person ...
3. *Coordinated Care:* ... coordinates care across all elements of the broader health care system, including specialty care, hospitals, home health care, and community services and supports ...
4. *Accessible Services:* ... delivers accessible services with shorter waiting times for urgent needs, enhanced in-person hours, around-the-clock telephone or electronic access to a member of the care team, and alternative methods of communication such as email and telephone care ...
5. *Quality and Safety:* ... demonstrates a commitment to quality and quality improvement by ongoing engagement

in activities such as using evidence-based medicine and clinical decision-support tools to guide shared decision making with patients and families, engaging in performance measurement and improvement, measuring and responding to patient experiences and patient satisfaction, and practicing population health management ..."[34]

PEARL

A traditional medical education term, "Clinical Pearls" refer to key patient care points, critical concepts and actions (in other words, the bullet points of patient care).

Population Health Management (PHM; Population Health) Since entering the healthcare lexicon in 2003, "Population Health Management" has multiplied and evolved into "Population Medicine," "Population Health," "Population Management," and other related terms so that today, there is no uniform definition.[35] That said, whether focused on outcomes, measures, payment, and/or accountability (or some other metric), PHM represents a major shift from the focus on the individual patient and the individual doctor-patient relationship to management/care of populations of individuals grouped based upon similar, addressable characteristics (clinical and/or nonclinical).

PQRS "The Physician Quality Reporting System (PQRS) is a quality reporting program that ... [requires] individual ... [providers] and group practices to report information on the quality of care to Medicare."[36] The PQRS System is utilized in Medicare reimbursement decisions (that is, failing to meet these government-specified quality outcomes can result in financial penalization).

Preventable Medical Error Exactly as it sounds: an error in patient care that is preventable if appropriate current, credible, evidence-based information and guidance and/or appropriate clinical skills are utilized.

Primary Care Physician (PCP) Believe it or not, there are varying definitions of a primary care physician (legal, operational, reimbursement, and other). The Patient Protection and Affordable Care Act (ACA) defines a PCP as "a physician who has a primary specialty designation of family medicine, internal medicine, geriatric medicine, or pediatric medicine."[37] Legally, a PCP is defined as "a physician or medical doctor specializing either in internal medicine, pediatric medicine or family or general practice, providing both first hand care for a person with undiagnosed health concern and continuing care for patients with varied medical conditions."[38] (Of note, today's reform is expanding the definition to include *non-physician* primary care provider, with the verbiage evolving into "Primary Care *Practitioner,* or PCP.")

Reference Solutions The classic example of a clinical decision support *pull* solution (a CDS tool which requires the user to know what they wish to search for and to actively seek the information and guidance), reference solutions range from textbooks and journals to websites and advanced information resources integrated into an HIT network. The critical distinction between differing reference solutions is whether the solution sources are *current, credible,* and *evidence-based,* all necessary in today's healthcare reform environment.

Signs and Symptoms Regularly confused by non-clinicians (and even by some clinicians), *there is a very clear clinical distinction between these two terms.* Symptoms represent a *patient's subjective complaints and feelings* (such as belly pain or skin redness). Symptoms often guide the clinician's initial diagnostic evaluation plan. Signs are *objective evidence of pathology* (such as abdominal tenderness to palpation or skin erythema and blanching) and are often even more beneficial in directing the diagnostic process. In simplest terms, symptoms are "what the patient feels," and signs are "what the provider finds."

The Triple Aim Developed by the Institute for Healthcare Improvement, The Triple Aim "is a framework … that describes an approach to optimizing health system performance. … to simultaneously pursue three dimensions …

- Improving the patient experience of care (including quality and satisfaction);
- Improving the health of populations; and
- Reducing the per capita cost of health care."[39]

The Triple Aim has been adopted by the US government (and numerous private entities as well as nations outside of the United States) as a high-level roadmap to improved health and reduced costs of care.

Technology Informatics Guiding Education Reform (TIGER) Initiative "TIGER is a grassroots initiative focused on education reform and interprofessional community development. The spirit of TIGER is to maximize the integration of technology and informatics into seamless practice, education and research resource development."[40] TIGER is definitely interprofessional by design, and there are numerous opportunities for providers from all disciplines to participate in this initiative.

Tort Reform There are multiple flavors of proposed healthcare tort reform, but the term generally refers to the modification of our legal system to increase the difficulty ("raise the bar") for those wishing to bring suit against one or more providers (including provider organizations) for malpractice, and/or to reduce the maximum financial awards to be paid by provider defendants as a result of successful malpractice litigation. Many people feel strongly that tort reform would significantly decrease US healthcare costs by reducing the pressure on providers to practice defensive medicine and by decreasing the number of frivolous lawsuits filings. (In fact, many argue that the absence of tort reform in the Patient Protection and Affordable Care Act limits the legislation's potential to significantly reduce healthcare spending.) Those opposed to or concerned about tort reform argue that if overly aggressive, patients who are truly harmed by clearly negligent care will find it too difficult to sue the responsible providers and, even if successful, the awards received may be inappropriately low relative to the preventable injury suffered.

US National Health Expenditure This is the US government's official measure of spending on all healthcare goods and services over a specified period of time (think of it as analogous to the gross domestic product specific to the healthcare sector).

Value-Based Care The foundation of the current healthcare reform revolution, value-based care targets the consistent delivery of high quality, cost-efficient patient care (quality being the numerator in the value equation and cost being the denominator). In lay terms, value-based care is in direct opposition to the traditional American healthcare system, in which neither the quality nor the cost of care are uniformly accepted major care metrics.

Value-Based Reimbursement The driving force behind value-based care, value-based reimbursement is the provider payment model at the heart of current healthcare reform. Unlike the fee-for-service model, in which reimbursement is unrelated to quality or cost-efficiency of the care delivered, the relationship between value and payment is the basis of value-based reimbursement. Through legislated federal programs, providers are eligible to share in any savings when meeting government-specified quality outcomes through cost-efficient care delivery. However, this "carrot" has been perceived as relatively small and extremely difficult to attain. The "stick," however, is much larger and comes in the form of significant Medicare reimbursement penalties for quality outcomes falling below the government-specified levels. It is the threat of these value-based reimbursement penalties that are driving the challenging pace of HIT purchasing activities by provider organizations across the nation (and which, unfortunately, often allow too little time for thoughtful, strategic discussion prior to action).

Workflow Solutions "Workflow is the sequence of physical and mental tasks performed by various people within and between work environments. … For example, the workflow of ordering a medication includes communication between the provider and the patient, the provider's thought process, the physical action by the provider of writing a paper prescription or entering an electronic prescription into an electronic health record and transmitting the order electronically or having the patient take the prescription to the pharmacy to have the prescription filled."[41] In other words, your workflow describes all of the thoughts, decisions, activities, and actions that you create and/or implement and that impact you (from outside sources) during your daily patient care activities.

References

1. Neporent L. Obamacare Explained (Like You're an Idiot). *ABC News (online)*. 2013; http://abcnews.go.com/Health/obamacare-explained-idiot/story?id=21292932.
2. Accountable Care Organizations (ACOs): General Information. CMS.gov (online) 2017; https://innovation.cms.gov/initiatives/aco/.
3. Centers for Disease Control and Prevention (online) 2014; https://www.cdc.gov/maso/pdf/cdcmiss.pdf.
4. Clinical Decision Support. Agency for Healthcare Research and Quality (online) 2014; https://www.ahrq.gov/professionals/prevention-chronic-care/decision/clinical/index.html.
5. Eligible Professional Meaningful Use Core Measures. CMS.gov (online) 2014; https://www.cms.gov/Regulations-and-Guidance/Legislation/EHRIncentivePrograms/downloads/1_CPOE_for_Medication_Orders.pdf.
6. Medical Definition of Defensive Medicine. MedicineNet.com (online) 2016; http://www.medicinenet.com/script/main/art.asp?articlekey=33262.
7. Evidence-Based Practice in Psychology. American Psychological Association (online) 2017; http://www.apa.org/practice/resources/evidence/.
8. Woodbury G and Kuhnke J. Evidence-based practice vs. evidence-informed practice: what's the difference? *Research Gate* (online) 2014; https://www.researchgate.net/publication/260793333_Evidence-based_Practice_vs_Evidence-informed_Practice_What%27s_the_Difference.
9. What Is an Electronic Health Record (EHR)? HealthIT.gov (online) 2013; https://www.healthit.gov/providers-professionals/faqs/what-electronic-health-record-ehr.

10. Garrett P. *EMR vs EHR—What is the Difference? HealthITBuzz* (online); 2011. https://www.healthit. gov/buzz-blog/electronic-health-and-medical-records/ emr-vs-ehr-difference/.

11. Groundless Many Malpractice Cases. *NBC News* (online); 2006. http://www.nbcnews.com/id/12723303/ns/health-health_care/t/many-medical-malpractice-cases-groundless/#. WOug-GcpCpo.

12. A Brief Guide to Genomics. NIH National Human Genome Research Institute (online) 2015; https://www.genome. gov/18016863/.

13. Measuring the Economy: A Primer on GDP and the National Income and Product Accounts. *Bureau of Economic Analysis, U.S Department of Commerce* (online) 2015; https://bea.gov/ NATIONAL/PDF/NIPA_PRIMER.PDF.

14. Koba M. Gross Domestic Product: CNBC Explains. *CNBC (online)*. 2011;. http://www.cnbc.com/id/44505017.

15. Basics of Health IT. HealthIT.gov (online) 2013; https://www. healthit.gov/patients-families/basics-health-it.

16. Health Information Technology. HHS.gov (online); https:// www.hhs.gov/hipaa/for-professionals/special-topics/health-information-technology/index.html.

17. Health Literacy. U.S. Department of Health and Human Services, Health Resources and Services Administration (online) 2016; https://www.hrsa.gov/publichealth/healthliteracy/.

18. HIMSS (online) 2017; http://www.himss.org/.

19. Health IT Legislation and Regulations. HealthIT. gov (online) 2016; https://www.healthit.gov/ policy-researchers-implementers/health-it-legislation.

20. Hospital Consumer Assessment of Healthcare Providers and Systems (online) (n.d.); http://hcahpsonline.org/home.aspx.

21. HCAHPS: Patients' Perspectives of Care Survey. CMS. gov (online) 2014; https://www.cms.gov/Medicare/ Quality-Initiatives-Patient-Assessment-Instruments/ HospitalQualityInits/HospitalHCAHPS.html.

22. Institute for Healthcare Improvement (online) 2017; http:// www.ihi.org/about/Pages/default.aspx.

23. Sheet Post-Acute Care Cheat. Integrated Delivery Networks. *Advisory Board* (online). 2014; https://www.advisory.com/ research/post-acute-care-collaborative/members/resources/ cheat-sheets/integrated-delivery-networks.

24. Core Competencies for Interprofessional Collaborative Practice. Interprofessional Education Collaborative (online) 2011; http://www.aacn.nche.edu/education-resources/ IPECReport.pdf.

25. Bal SB. An introduction to medical malpractice in the United States. *Clin Orthop Relat Res*. 2009;467:339–347.

26. Meaningful Use Definition and Objectives. HealthIT. gov (online) 2015; https://www.healthit.gov/ providers-professionals/meaningful-use-definition-objectives.

27. Medicaid.gov (online) 2017; https://www.medicaid.gov/ medicaid/index.html.

28. Medicare. USA.gov (online) 2017; https://www.usa.gov/ medicare/.

29. About ONC. HealthIT.gov (online) 2016; https://www.healthit. gov/newsroom/about-onc.

30. Outpatient and Ambulatory Surgery CAHPS (OAS CAHPS). CMS.gov (online) 2016; https://www.cms.gov/Research-Statistics-Data-and-Systems/Research/CAHPS/OAS-CAHPS.html.

31. Ambulatory Surgery Center Association (online) (n.d.); http://www.ascassociation.org/federalregulations/qualityreporting/oascahpssurveyfaqs.

32. Institute for Healthcare Improvement (online) 2017; http://www.ihi.org/Topics/TripleAim/Pages/Overview.aspx.

33. Stanton, MW. Expanding Patient-Centered Care To Empower Patients and Assist Providers Research in Action. *U.S. Department of Health and Human Services, Agency for Healthcare Research and Quality* (online) 2002;(5). https://archive.ahrq.gov/research/findings/factsheets/patient-centered/ria-issue5/ria-issue5.html.

34. Defining the PCMH. U.S. Department of Health and Human Services, Agency for Healthcare Research and Quality (online) 2014; https://pcmh.ahrq.gov/page/defining-pcmh.

35. Defining Pizzi R, Health Population. *Healthcare IT News* (online); 2015. http://www.healthcareitnews.com/blog/defining-population-health.

36. Physician Quality Reporting System. CMS.gov (online) 2016; https://www.cms.gov/Medicare/Quality-Initiatives-Patient-Assessment-Instruments/PQRS/index.html.

37. CMS Manual System. *Department of Health & Human Services, Centers for Medicare & Medicaid Services* (online) 2011; https://www.cms.gov/Regulations-and-Guidance/Guidance/Transmittals/downloads/R2161CP.pdf.

38. Primary Care Physician (PCP) Law and Legal Definition. US Legal (online) 2016; https://definitions.uslegal.com/p/primary-care-physician-pcp/.

39. The IHI Triple Aim. Institute for Healthcare Improvement (online) 2017; http://www.ihi.org/engage/initiatives/TripleAim/Pages/default.aspx.

40. The TIGER Initiative. HIMSS (online) 2017; http://www.himss.org/professionaldevelopment/tiger-initiative.

41. What Is Workflow? *U.S. Department of Health and Human Services, Agency for Healthcare Research and Quality* (online) 2014; https://healthit.ahrq.gov/health-it-tools-and-resources/workflow-assessment-health-it-toolkit/workflow.

INDEX

Page numbers followed by *f* indicate figures and *b* indicate boxes.